16 MYTHS OF A DIABETIC DIET

SECOND EDITION

Karen Hanson Chalmers, MS, RD, LDN, CDE
Amy Peterson Campbell, MS, RD, LDN, CDE

American Diabetes Association.
Cure • Care • Commitment®

Director, Book Publishing, Robert Anthony; *Managing Editor, Book Publishing,* Abe Ogden; *Editor,* Greg L. Guthrie; *Production Manager,* Melissa Sprott; *Composition,* American Diabetes Association; *Cover Design,* Jody Billert/Design Literate, Inc.; *Printer,* United Graphics Incorporated.

Printed in the United States of America

1 3 5 7 9 10 8 6 4 2

ADA titles may be purchased for business or promotional use or for special sales. To purchase more than 50 copies of this book at a discount, or for custom editions of this book with your logo, contact Jewelyn Morris, Special Sales & Promotions, at the address below, or at JMorris@diabetes.org or 703-299-2085.

For all other inquiries, please call 1-800-DIABETES.

American Diabetes Association
1701 North Beauregard Street
Alexandria, Virginia 22311

Library of Congress Cataloging-in-Publication Data

Chalmers, Karen.
   16 myths of a diabetic diet / Karen Hanson Chalmers, Amy Peterson Campbell. — 2nd ed.
      p. cm.
   Includes index.
   ISBN 978-1-58040-287-3 (alk. paper)

   1. Diabetes—Diet therapy. 2. Medical misconceptions. I. Campbell, Amy Peterson, 1964- II. Title. III. Title: Sixteen myths of a diabetic diet.
   RC662.C45 2007
   616.4'620654—dc22

                              2007021343

To our patients, friends, and family members
with diabetes, who have taught us so much about
what it means to live with diabetes.

To my husband, Rob. As a person who has lived with diabetes
for more than 30 years, you're an inspiration and role model for
children and adults with diabetes. Thanks for all that you do.
—A.P.C.

To Kara, Nate, and Erin: You have all demonstrated
incredible strength, support, and courage during challenging
times. Thank you. To Gabriella: A strong and beautiful
gift who has brought joy into our lives.
—K.H.C.

CONTENTS

PREFACE...VII

INTRODUCTION 1

Chapter 1: MEDICAL NUTRITION THERAPY VERSUS
      THE DIABETIC DIET 5

Myth: *People with diabetes must eat only low-calorie foods and special foods from the "dietetic" section in the supermarket.*

Chapter 2: SUGAR 17

Myth: *People with diabetes must avoid all foods that contain sugar.*

Chapter 3: STARCH AND FIBER..29

Myth: *People with diabetes should avoid potatoes, pasta, rice, and bread because starchy foods raise blood glucose levels and cause weight gain.*

Chapter 4: PROTEIN 43

Myth: *People with diabetes should follow a high-protein diet to stay healthy and strong.*

Chapter 5: FAT 59

Myth: *People with diabetes have to follow a rigid fat-free diet.*

Chapter 6: SUGAR SUBSTITUTES...73

Myth: *People with diabetes should only eat sugar-free foods.*

Chapter 7: CARBOHYDRATE COUNTING AND
      THE GLYCEMIC INDEX..85

Myth: *People with diabetes must follow a diabetic diet that uses exchanges (or choices) to plan their meals.*

Chapter 8: LABEL READING 99

Myth: *People with diabetes need to only look at sugar and calories on food labels.*

Chapter 9: DIABETES AND BODY WEIGHT...........................117

Myth: *People with diabetes should lose a lot of weight in order to control their blood glucose levels.*

Chapter 10: DIABETES AND THE USE OF SUPPLEMENTS 135

Myth: *People with diabetes should take special dietary supplements.*

Chapter 11: SODIUM...151

Myth: *People with diabetes should be on a low-sodium diet.*

Chapter 12: SNACKS..165

Myth: *People with diabetes must eat a snack between meals and particularly at bedtime to prevent low blood glucose levels.*

Chapter 13: EXERCISE 177

Myth: *People with diabetes should exercise every day in order to stay healthy.*

Chapter 14: DINING OUT WITH DIABETES...........................193

Myth: *People with diabetes shouldn't eat out.*

Chapter 15: DIABETES AND FOOD CRAVINGS 205

Myth: *People with diabetes don't get food cravings.*

Chapter 16: MAKING FAVORITE RECIPES HEALTHIER 221

Myth: *People with diabetes should only use diabetic cookbooks and recipes.*

Appendix A: "YOUR TURN" ANSWER KEY 237

Appendix B: REGISTERED DIETITIANS
            AND CERTIFIED DIABETES EDUCATORS 241

INDEX..247

PREFACE

As a person with long-standing type 1 diabetes (almost 54 years at this writing), I have learned a good deal about this disease over the years. My information has come from doctors, nurse educators, dietitians, family members, and friends. It has come in the form of books, conversations, magazine articles, and, more recently, online articles. And it has come from practicing the art of living with diabetes. Probably the most important thing I have learned in all this time is that I can always learn more.

When I was diagnosed at the tender age of four, diabetes care was very different than it is now. I was taught to categorize and weigh all of my foods (carbs, proteins, and fats alike) by my father, a scientist and professor. He and my mother learned all they could from my doctor at the Joslin Diabetes Center in Boston, Dr. Priscilla White. In addition to diet planning and measuring, our tools included metal and glass syringes with separate metal needles that regularly became dull. My father tested the needles on his thigh as he sharpened them! All the injection equipment had to be kept in a special sterile bath between uses. My parents, and soon I, tested my urine for sugar several times a day using an eye dropper and a tablet that boiled and changed colors in the test tube. In short, we had none of the wonderfully liberating tools of today: glucose monitors, insulin pumps, glucose sensors, carbohydrate counting, the glycemic index, detailed food labels, and a half-century of research and studies aimed at understanding and improving our lives.

I first heard some of the diet myths described in this book when I was in my early twenties, while I attended a class at the Joslin Diabetes Center. Among the students were a number of newly diagnosed patients. I answered their numerous questions and misconceptions with what I hoped were accurate, even encouraging, anecdotes of my own struggles to balance food with insulin and with energy output (both physical and mental). I was horrified to learn that some people believed I could not eat anything with sugar in it! I have always loved fruits and vegetables and could not imagine living without them, let alone without the many varieties of rice, pasta, potatoes, corn, breads, and the occasional ice cream or cookie. I remember the mother of a five-year-old child asking me whether her daughter could ever again live a "normal" life and eat "normal" food. I hope she learned from the classes (and perhaps from me) that she not only *could* live a long, healthy, "normal" life, but most likely would.

Through the years I have encountered people living in the "diabetes Paleolithic" period, as I call it. They seem to carry the remnants of a genetic memory of a time before insulin was discovered and when having type 1 or "juvenile" diabetes was a death warrant: you could eat no carbohydrate because it would raise your blood sugar, which, without insulin, would slowly take away your life; therefore, starvation caused your early demise instead. It wasn't a pleasant choice, obviously. Comments from these "diabetes dinosaurs," such as, "Oh, you're diabetic? My grandmother died of that. She ate too much sugar," always sent me into training mode, and I would carefully explain how sugars are a natural part of many foods that we can and should eat, how we have to measure our food intake against our insulin doses and exercise, and how life with diabetes is a balancing act rather than a process of restriction or denial. Sometimes, the person listened politely, and I could almost see the information trickling out the other ear!

But for every diabetes dinosaur I have met, I have known several modern-day creatures: people who are genuinely interested in the subject, open minded, and pleased to ask questions and to learn more about life with diabetes. I hope you are that kind of person—with or without diabetes—because Amy Campbell and Karen Chalmers have here presented a wealth of information to live by. Their presentation is conversational, well organized, and chock full of comforting facts about eating healthfully. *16 Myths of a Diabetic Diet* is meant for people with newly diagnosed diabetes, those who have had it for decades, and their families, friends, and neighbors—in fact, for everyone who likes to eat.

Cynthia M. Shaler
Boalsburg, PA

INTRODUCTION

People with diabetes have identified "diet" as one of the most difficult parts of managing their condition. The word "diet" simply means "the food we eat to nourish our bodies." Diet is important to all people because the way you nourish your body affects growth and development, influences how you prevent and fight disease, and dictates your weight, energy level, and how you feel every day. Unfortunately, over the years, the term "diet" seems to have taken on a different meaning, particularly for those with diabetes. Currently, there are many misconceptions and a lot of negativity associated with the term.

The term diabetic diet has been around for centuries, dating as far back as 1550 B.C. Fortunately, since then many positive changes have taken place in nutrition science as it relates to diabetes. From the earliest treatment using rigidly controlled, semi-starvation diets to the "all foods can fit" thinking at the beginning of the 21st century, we have now arrived at nutrition science as we know it today, a science we call medical nutrition therapy.

Today, more and more people are being diagnosed with diabetes. For many, their first thoughts and questions usually center on food: "What can I eat?", "What foods should I avoid?", "How much can I eat?", "Do I have to give up all of my favorite foods?", "Am I always going to feel restricted?" The list goes on and on. Today, more and more people with diabetes are seeking a registered dietitian's care and counseling so that they can update their knowledge about food and diabetes and develop a realistic and individualized meal plan, together with their dietitian, to ensure healthy eating. Learning about current research and how it relates to food is essential for managing your diabetes.

Here are some of the facts you will learn when you meet with a registered dietitian:

- Food that is good for you is the same food that is good for the whole family!
- You can fit foods that contain sugar into your daily intake—you do not have to give up your favorite foods!
- You can eat a wide choice of foods—variety in meal planning is "in," restriction of foods is "out."
- Standardized "diabetic diets" are a thing of the past.
- Special "diet" foods are not needed—all foods can fit!
- Fats are now categorized as "healthy" or "unhealthy," and avoiding all fat is not the best option.
- Registered dietitians provide meal-planning options that are individualized and realistic, based on what you are willing and able to do.
- Moderate weight loss can result in improved blood sugar control and reaching an "ideal" body weight is not necessary.
- Eliminating carbohydrate from your diet and eating large amounts of protein is not a good substitute for healthy eating and weight loss.
- Snacks between meals and at bedtime are optional and certain types of foods work best to achieve satiety.
- Special vitamins and minerals are not needed for people with diabetes.
- Exercise does not have to involve a gym and spandex!

- Creating a plan before dining out can help you choose healthy options that are available at most restaurants.
- Old family recipes can be modified to make them lower in fat, carbohydrate, sodium, and calories.

One of the most important messages offered by your diabetes team is how to fit diabetes into your lifestyle rather than fitting your lifestyle into your diabetes. An important part of doing that is through learning the updated facts about healthy food choices for you and your family. We hope this book will serve as an important resource where you can find the most current information and research about nutrition and diabetes. Explore the 16 most common misconceptions about a diabetic diet—the first being that there even is such a thing! Moving beyond these myths is the best way to ensure the best management of your diabetes and ensure that you continue to enjoy the pleasures of the table.

CHAPTER 1

MEDICAL NUTRITION THERAPY VERSUS THE DIABETIC DIET

MYTH

People with diabetes must eat only low-calorie foods and special foods from the "dietetic section" in the supermarket.

NATE: My family doesn't understand that I can't eat the same meals that they eat because I now have diabetes! There are so many foods that I need to avoid, and I feel restricted and limited with my food choices!

DIETITIAN: Why do you think you have to avoid many foods and only eat "special foods" when you have diabetes?

NATE: My cousin, who has had diabetes for 20 years, told me he can't eat any foods with fat or sugar and that I should stay away from my family's favorite staple foods such as pasta and bread. I tried some of those "diabetic foods" but they are so expensive and the flavor isn't the same.

DIETITIAN: I'm happy that you came to see me today. I am confident that I can clear up a lot of the misconceptions that you and your family may have about diabetes and food. It's not uncommon for many people to think of a diabetic diet as lists of foods labeled "good" and "bad," while avoiding desserts and "sugar" foods. That is not how meal planning for people with diabetes works today. To put it simply, it is not about restriction! A person with diabetes can eat anything a person without diabetes eats, as long as he or she thinks about what they eat in terms of healthy eating and has accurate up-to-date education. The American Diabetes Association's goals for healthy eating aim at reducing fat and calories, including healthy carbohydrate foods, increasing fiber, moderating your protein intake, limiting alcohol intake, and fitting in regular physical activity. This is what anyone should be striving for—not just people with diabetes.

NATE: Do you really mean that I can continue to eat the foods that my family and I enjoy with just a little bit of tweaking?

DIETITIAN: Of course! There are no foods that are off limits, although some food choices are healthier than others. My job is to teach you to eat normally, but healthfully, so you can maintain your energy and blood glucose levels and understand how foods affect your blood glucose and weight. At the same time, doing this will help lower your risks of heart disease, high blood pressure, and kidney disease.

NATE: When can we start? I can't wait to begin eating like a "normal person" again.

WHAT'S NEXT?

There continues to be much confusion and debate about what foods to eat when you have diabetes. "What can I eat?" is the most often asked question, and Nate's thinking about a rigid "diabetic diet" and "forbidden foods" is all too common. Nate soon discovered that the "diet" for healthy living is based on flexible meal planning. Because his family was also at an increased risk of developing diabetes, such a meal plan would be helpful for them, too. What Nate perceived as a major challenge is now nothing more than learning how to enjoy his favorite foods balanced with new foods and that all foods can be part of a balanced diet.

THE OLD AND THE NEW

You may recall family members and friends describing nutrition guidelines for people with diabetes as being inflexible and tedious. To control blood glucose levels, doctors and dietitians had to provide strict, standardized "diabetic diets" to all people with diabetes. This diabetic diet was rigid and limited and distributed calories from carbohydrate, protein, and fat based on scientific research available at that time, which is now out of date. The biggest restriction, however, was the strict avoidance of sugar endorsed by a diabetic diet. Foods with added sugar, such as dessert foods, were prohibited, and even the amount of fruit, vegetables, and milk, which contained natural sugar, was severely regulated. People with diabetes often lost their motivation to stick with these preplanned diets, and their interest in nutrition diminished. Furthermore, the primary goal for blood glucose management back then was to reach an ideal body weight based on height and frame size.

Current nutrition guidelines are flexible and offer a wide variety of food choices. What was once a rigidly controlled, semi-starvation diet in the early days is now the "all foods can fit" meal plan that is tailor made for each person's food likes and dislikes, lifestyle, health risks, and diabetes medications. The "all foods can fit" motto balances food intake for people with diabetes and is now called *medical nutrition therapy* instead of a "diabetic diet." Health experts are no longer convinced that achieving an ideal body weight is a primary goal for managing your diabetes. Instead, you may be encouraged to maintain a reasonable weight or strive for a weight that you and your health care provider feel is realistic and achievable. We now know that even a moderate weight loss of 10–20 pounds for those who are overweight can result in improved blood glucose and blood fat levels.

As you read over the American Diabetes Association's medical nutrition therapy goals below, keep in mind that the 2005 U.S. Department of Agriculture (USDA) dietary guidelines for Americans and the American Heart Association recommendations are also very similar. Don't forget that these are guidelines for *all* healthy Americans.

> ## Summary of the 2006 American Diabetes Association's Updated Medical Nutrition Therapy (MNT) Recommendations
>
> People with diabetes should
> - receive individualized nutrition education, preferably provided by a registered dietitian who is a diabetes educator
> - make lifestyle changes, including weight loss, reduced fat intake, and regular physical activity
> - increase their daily fiber intake
> - minimize trans-fat and saturated fat intake
> - monitor carbohydrate intake to regulate blood glucose levels
> - limit daily alcohol intake

HERE ARE THE FACTS

The American diet clearly has *too much* fat, cholesterol, and sodium and *too little* fiber and healthy carbohydrates. Your overall health reflects many things, such as your environment, heredity, and regular health care. These are things that you do not always have complete control over. However, your food choices, which are controllable, can help you improve your health. Take a look at the following Dietary Guidelines for Americans:

Eat a variety of foods—diabetes still requires the same nutrients, vitamins, and minerals as for those without diabetes.

Maintain a healthy weight—excess body fat makes it more difficult to use insulin, which in turn can lead to high blood glucose levels.

Choose a diet low in total fat, trans-fat, saturated fat, and cholesterol—diabetes increases the risk for heart and blood vessel disorders.

Choose a diet with plenty of fresh vegetables, fruits, and whole-grain products—high fiber can help lower blood glucose and blood fat levels.

Use sugars only in moderation—with 16 calories per teaspoon, sugar is not particularly fattening, but many high-sugar foods contain less fiber and a lot of added fat that does contribute to weight gain.

Use salt and sodium in moderation—high blood pressure is common among people with diabetes, and too much salt may cause water retention.

If you drink alcoholic beverages, do so in moderation—alcohol can affect blood glucose and blood fat levels, as well as supply a lot of "empty calories."

DESIGNING YOUR OWN EATING PLAN

You will be happy to learn that registered dietitians offer a positive message that emphasizes the importance of healthy eating and daily physical activity. With the help of a registered dietitian, you'll be taught how to include foods you like to eat in your meal plan, identify what food groups these foods belong in, and make the best choices in quantity and quality for good health. You do not have to restrict foods that are high in fat, cholesterol, sugar, and sodium completely, but you do have to watch them. It is your overall intake of these foods over time that makes a difference, not a single food or meal. In the course of a day, it is important to know which foods are in each food group and the suggested food amounts from each food group.

The amount of food you should eat in a day depends on your age, gender, weight, and level of physical activity. Together with a registered dietitian, you will work to design an eating plan just for you that provides healthy calorie sources while still allowing you to eat many of your favorite foods. You will be assured of enough good sources of fiber and healthy carbohydrates and of how to cut down on the more unhealthy sources of fat, cholesterol, and sodium.

However, the most important point to remember is that actual "serving sizes" are usually smaller than what you are used to seeing on your plate. Instead of regularly eating smaller homemade meals, many Americans eat more restaurant meals and convenience foods, which provide larger portions than the standardized portion sizes found in *Choose Your Foods: Exchange Lists for Diabetes*. As these large portions become more familiar to us, portion sizes on our plates continue to grow bigger.

Let's briefly review the actual serving sizes of some common foods. These portion sizes are standardized and apply to all Americans, not just those with diabetes.

WHAT COUNTS AS ONE SERVING?

Carbohydrate

Including bread, cereals, grains, dry beans, crackers, snacks, and desserts.

- 1 slice bread
- 1/2 cup potato
- 1/2 cup cooked cereal
- 1 cup regular cereal

- 1/2 cup corn or peas
- 1/2 cup lentils or beans
- 1/3 cup pasta or rice
- 1 low-fat granola bar
- 1/4 large bagel (1 oz)
- 3 cups air-popped popcorn
- 2 rice cakes
- 1/2 cup low-fat ice cream

Fruits and Vegetables

- 1 small fresh fruit
- 1/2 cup canned fruit or juice
- 1 cup berries
- 17 grapes
- 1/2 grapefruit
- 1/4 cup dried fruit
- 1 cup raw vegetables
- 1/2 cup cooked vegetables
- 1/2 cup vegetable juice

Milk and Yogurt

- 1 cup nonfat or low-fat milk
- 6 oz nonfat or low-fat yogurt
- 1 cup sugar-free cocoa
- 1 cup low-fat soy/rice milk
- 1/3 cup dry low-fat milk

Protein

Including meat and meat substitutes.
- 1 oz lean fish, meat, or poultry
- 1 oz low-fat cheese
- 1 egg

- 1/4 cup egg substitute
- 1/4 cup low-fat cottage cheese
- 2 oz tofu
- 2 Tbsp natural peanut butter

Fat

- 1 tsp butter/margarine
- 1 Tbsp lite margarine
- 1 Tbsp salad dressing
- 1 tsp oil
- 1 tsp mayonnaise
- 1 Tbsp light mayonnaise
- 6 almonds/cashews
- 1 Tbsp sunflower seeds
- 2 Tbsp light sour cream/cream cheese

Alcohol

- 1 1/2 oz liquor
- 12 oz lite beer
- 5 oz dry wine

Variables

Now that you have reviewed the appropriate serving sizes of some common foods, it is important to note that you may eat more than one serving. For example, a dinner portion of meat (protein) for a young, active male could be five to six servings (5–6 oz), whereas a dinner portion for a middle-aged, non-active woman may be two to three servings (2–3 oz). This is all determined by working together with a registered dietitian who can personalize a meal plan to meet your specific needs. If you have type 2 diabetes and control your diabetes by diet and exercise alone, or in combination with diabetes medications, you may be asked to eat consistent amounts of carbohydrate at meals as well as regulate the timing of your meals to coincide with the action of your diabetes medication(s). If you have type 1 or type 2 diabetes and are on insulin, you may be asked to eat a consistent amount of carbohydrate at meals or you may learn how to precisely match your insulin to the amount of carbohydrate you plan to eat for more flexibility. So, there are certain considerations that should be taken into account depending on the type of medication you are on for your diabetes as well as how your specific insulin dose is calculated at each meal.

HERE'S WHAT YOU CAN DO

1. **You are a normal, healthy person who just happens to have diabetes.** Don't think of your diabetes as a disorder that takes all of the pleasure and taste out of eating. Remember, there are no foods that are off limits.

2. **Get help.** Sit down with a registered dietitian to find out where most of your calories are coming from. Are you eating too many fat-filled and animal foods and not enough whole grains, fruits, and vegetables? Have you eliminated carbohydrate foods from your diet? What do you need to eat more of? What do you need to eat less of?

3. **Eat a variety of fresh fruits and vegetables every day.**

4. **Eat fewer animal products.** Doing this will reduce your risk of heart disease.

5. **Eat more fiber.** Choose whole-grain breads and cereals. Eat the skins and peels of fresh fruits and vegetables. Add dried beans and lentils.

6. **Eat less fat.** Try to cut down on trans-fats and saturated fats, which are harmful to your arteries.

7. **Cut down on your salt intake.** Cut down on the salt you use when cooking and at the table.

8. **Make a healthy grocery shopping list.** Be sure to include more of the foods you have been missing and make an effort to include these foods on a regular basis.

9. **Get help with weight loss.** If you are trying to lose weight, let your registered dietitian help you tighten up your portion sizes and increase activity. Doing this will allow you to eat fewer calories and burn more calories.

10. **Use teamwork.** Work with your diabetes team and dietitian to coordinate your food intake with your activity level and diabetes medication(s).

11. **Plan on eating meals that fill you up for longer periods.** Such meals contain moderate amounts of protein and healthy fats and contain fiber-rich carbohydrate foods, such as whole-grain starches, fruits, and vegetables.

12. **Educate your family and support system.** Help your family members understand how to eat in a healthy way by bringing variety and balance from all of the food groups to your shared meals.

COMMONLY ASKED QUESTIONS

Will I still be able to keep good control of my blood glucose if I eat the same foods as the rest of the family?

If you work with your diabetes team and your registered dietitian to match your food intake with your diabetes medications and activity level, you won't have to eat any differently than the rest of your family, assuming they are also eating a healthy, balanced diet.

How can I make wise food choices to lower my risk for heart disease and other problems caused by diabetes?

Keep your blood glucose in your target range and stick with your healthful eating plan, regular physical activity, and, if needed, diabetes medications.

Isn't it more important for a person with diabetes to follow healthy eating guidelines than for the rest of the family?

Healthy eating guidelines are important for all Americans because we tend to eat too much fat, cholesterol, and sodium and not enough fiber and healthy carbohydrates. Because of excesses in our diets, all Americans are at a greater risk for heart disease, high blood pressure, stroke, diabetes, obesity or overweight, and some forms of cancer.

YOUR TURN

Now it's your turn to recall some key points from this chapter. Let's see how you do!

1. Instead of the term "diabetic diet," we now call meal planning for those with diabetes _____ (3 words).
2. Achieving a "reasonable body weight" rather than "ideal body weight" is now one of the primary goals for diabetes self-management. True or false?
3. Please fill out what counts as one standardized serving size, for each of the following foods:

   Rice/pasta: _____

   Cooked oatmeal: _____

   Lentils/beans: _____

   Berries: _____

   Milk: _____

   Light margarine/mayonnaise: _____

   Olive oil: _____
4. Currently, nutrition guidelines are flexible and offer a wide variety of food choices. True or false?

See APPENDIX A for the answers.

CHAPTER 2

SUGAR

> ## MYTH
>
> People with diabetes must avoid all foods that contain sugar.

JUDY: I was just diagnosed with diabetes right before moving to this area. My former doctor told me to stay away from any foods with sugar—I can't even eat carrots! She also told me to see a registered dietitian but didn't tell me how to find one.

DIETITIAN: You must be feeling completely over-whelmed by your new diagnosis. You must also feel very limited with your food choices. The good news is that the main goal of medical nutrition therapy for those with diabetes is not to avoid sugar, but to eat a healthy balance of foods spread out over the day.

JUDY: I remember that my grandmother had diabetes for years and could never eat desserts or foods with sugar. Even after depriving herself for years, she still had many complications related to diabetes. And to make matters worse, I'm addicted to sugar!

DIETITIAN: Actually, new nutrition guidelines were introduced by the American Diabetes Association in the 2000s. Each year, the nutrition guidelines are updated based on the most current research. So, not only can sugar be added into any healthy eating plan, but we now have many new treatment options for people with diabetes to prevent or delay the complications of diabetes. There are two other pieces of good news. One is that you can certainly eat carrots! The second is that although people do like and desire foods with sugar, this does not qualify as an addiction.

WHAT'S NEXT?

The need to avoid sugar is one of the biggest misconceptions in diabetes management today. Like Judy, many people with diabetes mistakenly work extremely hard to eliminate all foods with sugar. Judy learned that this was nearly an impossible task because many healthy foods have some form of sugar in them. Some foods contain "added sugars," whereas other foods naturally contain sugar. Many research studies completed over the past 30 years have shown that foods containing sugar can be part of a healthy diet, even for those people with diabetes, and can be fit into an eating plan, just like any other carbohydrate food.

After several diabetes appointments with the dietitian, Judy learned that sugar is not forbidden or harmful and began to feel more comfortable about fitting many new foods that contained sugar into her eating plan. Instead of feeling guilty about eating sugar and trying to avoid it at all costs, Judy was able to take control of her situation and manage to fit some foods with sugar into her eating plan.

THE OLD AND THE NEW

Nutrition therapy has always been the cornerstone in the self-management of diabetes; however, some people with diabetes have had little training in medical nutrition therapy and may have been told to "watch their diet" and to "stay away from sugar."

A brief historic review reveals that hundreds of years ago, diabetes was attributed to eating an excessive amount of food with sugar and flour. This meant that mostly all carbohydrate foods were restricted and that those with diabetes were put on a "starvation diet" of mostly fat and some protein. From that time, until insulin was discovered in 1921, a person's carbohydrate content came only from vegetables, such as onions, lettuce, radishes, cabbage, and mustard greens. Eventually, insulin was isolated in 1921, and the "starvation diet" took a giant step backward, while various nutritious food choices started taking baby steps forward. Although fruits were mostly restricted, carbohydrate intake was on the upswing, from 20% of calories from carbohydrate in 1921 to what the American Diabetes Association now recommends as that amount of carbohydrate based on each individual's blood glucose, weight, and lipid goals. However, it wasn't until the 1980s, when home blood glucose monitoring was introduced, that health professionals started to understand how certain carbohydrates really affected blood glucose levels.

For years, people with diabetes were taught to avoid *concentrated sweets*, known as *simple sugars*, because they were thought to overload the blood with sugar much faster than starches, which were known as complex carbohydrates. Dr. Elliot Joslin stated the general consensus about starch and sugar best in his early editions of *Joslin's Diabetic Manual for Doctor and Patient*:

- Sugar enters the blood as fast as a child runs.
- Starch enters the blood as fast as a child walks.
- Starch in vegetables enters the blood as slowly as a child creeps.

This was the explanation used when emphasizing to people with diabetes how important it was to strictly avoid sugar, to carefully measure starchy foods, and to eat vegetables more freely. We followed the assumption that sugar was harmful to people with diabetes until the

1970s, when scientists started to look for clear evidence of how sugar and diabetes interacted. In the latter part of the 20th century, the American Diabetes Association and prominent researchers in the field of diabetes studied the published findings from many scientific studies on nutrition and diabetes. They concluded that there was *little* scientific evidence to suggest that sugar is more quickly digested and absorbed into the bloodstream or that sugar elevates blood sugar more than starch. Sugar, we learned, has an impact on blood glucose similar to that of any other carbohydrate. Therefore, the use of sugar as part of the *total* carbohydrate content of the diet is okay for people with diabetes as long as these sugar-containing foods are substituted for other carbohydrate foods as part of a balanced meal plan. Nutrition therapy is no longer about *avoiding* sugar but rather about well-controlled blood glucose levels. Finally, people with diabetes started being taught how to eat *realistically* instead of *ideally*.

What Is Sugar?

The three types of carbohydrate are *sugar*, *starch*, and *fiber*. These carbohydrates are all made up of a certain number of "sugar blocks." Some are single blocks, some are double, and some are many blocks connected together in long chains. Carbohydrates do, however, vary in their chemical structure and in the number of units (or sugar blocks) that are put together to make them. The carbohydrates with only one or two sugar blocks are called *simple carbohydrates*. The carbohydrates with many sugar blocks connected together are called *complex carbohydrates* (see Chapter 3).

There are six important sugars in nutrition. Three are *single* sugars (monosaccharides) and three are *double* sugars (disaccharides).

The single sugar blocks are the *monosaccharides*: glucose, fructose, and galactose. The double sugar blocks are the *disaccharides*: maltose (glucose + glucose), sucrose (glucose + fructose), and lactose (glucose + galactose).

Starch and fiber are called polysaccharides and are composed of straight or branched chains of the single sugars called monosaccharides. In this chapter, we are mostly talking about sugars (or *simple carbohydrate*) because these are the carbohydrates that many people with diabetes think they have to avoid.

The Monosaccharides

Glucose is the largest, the most common, and the most complicated of all of the sugars. Glucose is always found as one of the two sugars in disaccharides and is the basic unit of starch and fiber. Glucose is simply the form that carbohydrate takes in the body as our fuel.

When carbohydrates are digested, they are converted into glucose and our blood sugar levels rise. Almost 100% of carbohydrate foods break down into glucose and are available as fuel. Therefore, carbohydrate is our main source of energy. We do not always use all of the blood sugar from carbohydrate right away. With insulin's help, some glucose is stored in the liver, where is it changed into a storage form of glucose called glycogen. This glycogen can give you quick energy if you should need it and takes care of your energy needs while you are sleeping. Fuel is also stored in muscle as glycogen, but this storage does not last long, especially during exercise.

Fructose is the sweetest of the sugars and, in combination with glucose, is a component of table sugar (sucrose). Fructose occurs naturally in fruits, berries, vegetables, and honey. It is also used as an additive in products sweetened with high-fructose corn syrup, a food additive that people with diabetes should cut down on. Although many people with diabetes believe fructose may be a better choice as a sweetener, the American Diabetes Association states that the "use of added fructose as a sweetening agent in the diabetic diet may have no overall advantage over other sweeteners."

Galactose is not as common as glucose and fructose. It is one of the three monosaccharides common in foods but its sugar block is always connected to another sugar block to form lactose, the sugar in milk.

The Disaccharides

The disaccharides are double sugar blocks of the three sugars above, with glucose being a part of all three sugars.

Maltose consists of two glucose units and is only a part of a few foods. Maltose appears when starch is broken down, such as during digestion, when seeds germinate, and when alcohol is fermented.

Sucrose consists of fructose and glucose and forms what we know as table sugar. This is the most common of all the sugars and gets its sweet taste from fructose. The main food sources of sucrose are the juice from sugar cane and sugar beets. Sucrose is processed to make brown, white, or powdered sugar. Today, sucrose can be part of an eating plan for *anyone* with diabetes. It is no longer forbidden or restricted for people with diabetes, although it should be used in moderation.

Lactose consists of galactose and glucose and is a disaccharide found in the milk of mammals. Lactose is the main carbohydrate found in milk and often referred to as milk sugar.

WHERE IS IT FOUND?

Natural or Added?

So now you know that sugar—any kind of sugar—is just a *type of carbohydrate* and is only one type of sugar among several that are found in foods. Although we now know that sugar has a similar impact on blood sugar as do many other carbohydrates, let's think about how sugar occurs in food: is it found *naturally* in food or is it *added* to the food? Natural or added sugars still have the same effect on blood sugar levels; however, the foods that contain these sugars may not be equally healthy or nutritious.

For instance, an apple contains carbohydrate in a *natural* sugar (fructose), whereas a candy bar contains its carbohydrate from an *added* sugar (sucrose). You know the apple is healthier because it is a good source of many vitamins, minerals, and fiber. The candy bar, on the other hand, is what we call an empty-calorie food, which means that although it may taste good, it doesn't offer any health benefits. It also contributes a great deal of fat and calories. Remember, though, that you can choose to occasionally have an *empty-calorie food* as long as you substitute that food for another carbohydrate food. This is because your body does not necessarily recognize the natural or added sugars, but instead reacts to the *total* amount of carbohydrate you have eaten.

Finding the Sugar

One way to find the sugars in food is to look at the **Nutrition Facts** on a food label, under the Sugar category. But generally, you should look at the grams of Total Carbohydrate instead. Here's why.

If you look in the ingredient list, the sugars in the product will be individually listed, but often listed under an alias that most consumers do not recognize as sugars. The sugar listed on the label could include any of the following:

Brown sugar	Honey
Confectioners' sugar	Invert sugar
	Lactose
Carob	Maltose
Corn syrup	Maple syrup
Dextrose	Molasses
Fructose	Sucrose
Galactose	Turbinado
Glucose	

Some sugars listed in the ingredient list, but not necessarily listed next to sugar on the upper part of the label, include the sugar alcohols—hydrogenated starch hydrolysate, sorbitol, mannitol, maltitol, isomalt, and xylitol. The manufacturer is not required to list these sugar alcohols on a food label unless the food product clearly states that the food is "sugar-free." These *may* be listed next to "Other" or "Sugar Alcohols," directly under "Sugar," or they may be found only in the ingredient list. However, *all* sugars must be added to the grams of Total Carbohydrate. So overall, it is more important to look at grams of Total Carbohydrate than the grams of Sugar.

Some of the foods listed below will give you an idea of what *one* serving of a "sugar" food can look like:

2-inch square brownie	1 Tbsp 100% fruit spread
1/2 cup nonfat chocolate milk	1/2 cup regular gelatin
2-inch square unfrosted cake	1 Tbsp regular syrup (no fat)
1/4 cup sherbet or sorbet	1 granola bar
2 Tbsp light syrup (no fat)	1/2 sweet roll or Danish
	1/2 cup light or regular ice cream
	2 sandwich cookies

WHY DO WE NEED IT?

We don't really need sugar; however, sugar is found in many healthy foods and it tastes good. Natural sugars, such as those found in fruit, vegetables, and milk, make up about one-half of the sugar intake in the U.S. Added sugars, such as those found in cookies, soda, cakes, and candy, make up the other half of our sugar intake.

THE UPSIDE AND THE DOWNSIDE OF SUGAR

Sugar has received bad press for many years. Aside from the sweet taste that sugar adds to food, the only proven information that we have about sugar is that it contributes to tooth decay if eaten in excessive amounts. But we also know that, if eaten in moderation, when blood sugar control and weight are maintained, sugar is not necessarily harmful to our health. Let's clear up some of the confusion about sugar by looking at the upside and the downside of this controversial carbohydrate.

The Downside

Extra calories

Many empty-calorie foods such as candy, cake, and ice cream give you fuel and pleasure but none of the benefits of vitamins, minerals, fiber, and protein. If you are taking in 15–20 grams of carbohydrate from a candy bar instead of from a piece of fruit, then you will not only be taking in more calories (from fat), but you are also trading a healthy food for a not-so-healthy food. Even the fat-free versions of many of these empty-calorie foods will give you extra calories, because food manufacturers have to add more carbohydrate (sugar and/or starch) to stabilize the product when the fat is removed. Therefore, dessert foods should not replace healthier foods on a regular basis, regardless of whether you have diabetes.

Small portion sizes

Often if you eat a food that has a lot of its carbohydrate coming from sugar, you may have to eat a smaller quantity. For example, *1 cup* of Cheerios contains about *22 grams* of total carbohydrate:

1 gram comes from sugar

3 grams come from fiber

18 grams come from starch

However, if you decide to eat *1 cup* of Frosted Cheerios instead of the regular Cheerios, you will get *25 grams* of total carbohydrate:

13 grams come from sugar

1 gram comes from fiber

11 grams come from starch

So, if you are taking in 30 grams of carbohydrate from a cereal, you could have about 1 3/4 cups of Cheerios but only 1 1/4 cups of the Frosted Cheerios. You can leave it up to your appetite to decide which one you want.

Dental caries (cavities)

The digestive process begins in the mouth as soon as we start chewing food. Both sugar and starch break down into glucose in the mouth and equally contribute to tooth decay. Bacteria in the mouth thrive on food and ferment the sugars in carbohydrate foods. During the fermentation process, the bacteria produce and leave behind an acid that eats away at tooth enamel. The whole decaying process actually depends on how long the food stays in the mouth. However, regular brushing and flossing along with limiting large amounts of sticky carbohydrate foods will help prevent dental cavities.

The Upside

Moderation is the key

When eaten in moderation, sugar does not cause health problems such as obesity, hyperactivity, diabetes, and heart disease. However, sugar can contribute to weight gain and obesity if eaten in excess. It has actually been documented that obese people eat less sugar than do thin people.

Sugar does have positive traits as an additive

Sugar serves as a food additive to enhance and balance flavor and aroma by adding color and texture (that brown, crusty texture in baked goods). Sugar also acts as a preservative by keeping foods fresh. It adds bulk to ice cream and baked goods, helps to retain air in light-textured products, balances acidity, and lowers the freezing point of foods. Sugar also softens acidity and prolongs shelf life.

HERE'S WHAT YOU CAN DO

1. **Use sugar as part of your total carbohydrate intake.** This does not mean that you should eat unlimited amounts of sugar or dessert foods, but rather eat these foods in *moderation*. Totally eliminating sugar is unnecessary and impossible.

2. **Reduce the amount of sugars and dessert foods in your diet,** whether you have diabetes or not. Relate the amount of these foods in your diet to your level of activity and exercise.

3. **Read food labels** to determine how much of that food's carbohydrate is coming from sugar and if the food is nutritious rather than just an empty-calorie food. For instance, instead of chocolate cookies, eat oatmeal cookies; instead of frosted cereals, eat plain-type cereals and add berries for sweetness.

4. **Use the Serving Size as your guide** when eating high-sugar foods. Most average-size cookies list one or two cookies as a serving size, whereas ice creams list 1/2 cup as a serving size. Most people eat at least twice as much.

5. **Be sensible, but enjoy your new food choices.** You are not "cheating" if you eat foods that have sugar in them as long as your meals are within the context of healthy eating, meaning that you balance those foods with your carbohydrate intake. You are not a bad person for enjoying all foods. You are a normal person who happens to have diabetes and who has to live in the real world.

SUMMARY

Although it has been many years since nutrition guidelines for diabetes have become more realistic, people with diabetes still believe that avoiding sugar is the main goal of nutrition therapy. After years of educating people with diabetes about the dangers of sugar and giving them lists of "good" and "bad" foods, we now know that sugar is just a form of carbohydrate. With proper education from a registered dietitian, you can learn how to choose your carbohydrates wisely.

Your Turn

Now it's your turn to recall some key points from this chapter. Let's see how you do!

1. Natural sugars found in fruits, vegetables, and milk make up about one-half of the sugar intake in the U.S. Added sugars such as those in cookies, soda, cakes, and candy make up the other half. True or false?

2. The primary naturally occurring sugar found in milk is called _____ and is often called milk sugar.

3. Three examples of "empty-calorie foods" include:

   _____

   _____

   _____

4. You are "cheating" on your meal plan if you eat foods that have added sugar in them. True or false?

See APPENDIX A for the answers.

CHAPTER 3

STARCH AND FIBER

MYTH

People with diabetes should avoid potatoes, pasta, rice, and bread because starchy foods raise blood glucose levels and cause weight gain.

FERN: I recently read an article that said Americans should be adding more fiber to their diets and that fiber was also good for blood sugar and weight control. I wanted to start doing this, but I found that most high-fiber foods are also high in carbohydrate. I ended up coming home from the store with my usual purchases. Should I cut out all of the starchy foods and only eat foods with fiber, like raw vegetables and salad?

DIETITIAN: Starches and fiber are recommended for *all* people—not just those with diabetes. There are a variety of whole-grain starches and other high-fiber foods to choose from, such as whole-wheat pasta instead of white pasta and brown or whole-grain rice instead of white rice. Therefore, whole grains and other carbohydrate foods with fiber, such as fruits and vegetables, should be the most abundant foods on your plate. I will show you how to increase your fiber intake so you will be meeting the current recommendations of 20–35 grams per day.

FERN: But I heard that carbohydrate foods, particularly starches, make you *gain* weight and are the main *cause* of diabetes—not sugar!

DIETITIAN: Starches and sugars do not cause diabetes, but weight gain may occur if an excessive amount of any food is eaten. Starch, sugar, and fiber are all types of carbohydrate. Carbohydrate is our main source of fuel, and we need to eat some with each meal. Unfortunately, many Americans eat excessive amounts of carbohydrate because they are not aware of the portion sizes that they are eating. For example, *one serving* of a whole-grain food could be 1/2 cup cooked oatmeal, 1/3 cup cooked whole-wheat pasta or whole-grain brown rice, one-half of a 100% whole-grain English muffin, or one slice of whole-grain bread. How often do people just eat one slice of bread? The carbohydrate from these foods can add up very quickly at a meal, especially when added to other carbohydrate foods.

FERN: But why are those high-fiber foods so high in carbohydrate?

DIETITIAN: Although fiber is a type of carbohydrate, it is considered "roughage," so it has little impact on blood glucose levels and provides minimal calories. Therefore, dietary fiber can be deducted from the grams of Total Carbohydrate on a food label. I will be teaching you how to read food labels today. It is important to eat these high-fiber foods every day because roughage helps you feel more full after a meal, helps lower your cholesterol levels, and keeps your digestive tract healthy.

FERN: Okay, I'm ready to learn how to buy healthier foods and begin to add more fiber to my meals. I will also be mindful that it's the quantity and quality of starches that's important.

WHAT'S NEXT?

Many people view starchy foods as "bad" foods and try to eliminate many of these foods from their daily intake. When these same people also think of sugar foods as "bad" foods, they end up eliminating many healthy food choices (carbohydrates) as well as good sources of fiber, vitamins, and minerals from their eating plan.

Fern learned from her dietitian that starch and sugar foods are just two of the three types of carbohydrate that belong in everyone's food plan. Fern also learned that many carbohydrate foods also contain the third type of carbohydrate called fiber, which is the "roughage" that whole grains, fruits, and vegetables provide. Eating the recommended amount of 20–35 grams of fiber per day instead of the average American intake of 10–14 grams per day provides enough fiber to feel satisfied and full after eating a meal without adding extra calories.

Fern's dietitian also taught her how to keep track of her carbohydrate intake with a meal-planning method called *carbohydrate counting* (Chapter 7). This meal-planning method gave Fern a carbohydrate allowance to spend at each meal and snack. Much to her surprise, Fern was able to incorporate many new and different foods into her meals. By monitoring how much carbohydrate and fiber she was eating throughout the day, she not only was able to improve her blood glucose levels, but also found it easier to control her weight and food cravings by adding fiber-rich foods. Fern's last A1C revealed a significant improvement from her previous A1C.

THE OLD AND THE NEW

Before insulin was discovered in 1921, rigid restriction of carbohydrate foods was the only means of controlling blood sugar levels. However, a very small amount of carbohydrate coming from *fiber* was allowed in certain foods.

Foods were divided into categories based on the amount of carbohydrate and fiber they included. Vegetables such as lettuce, cucumbers, spinach, asparagus, celery, and cabbage were allowed in unlimited quantities. In *Joslin's Diabetic Manual for Doctor and Patient*, Dr. Elliot Joslin stated, "These vegetables are a comfort to a diabetic because they contain so little carbohydrate that they can be eaten freely, they are satisfying because of their bulk, and they are rich in vitamins A, B, and C." The next category included pumpkin, turnip, squash, beets, carrots, onions, and very young, fresh green peas. Then, more mature vegetables such as peas, lima beans, and parsnips were added in limited amounts. The last category was only to be used with caution. Foods such as potatoes, corn, bread, rice, macaroni, and beans were only allowed in very small quantities and had to be carefully measured.

With the discovery of insulin, carbohydrate in the form of starch was gradually increased to a small percentage of the total daily calories, although sugar in most forms, including many fruits, was still forbidden.

Over the next 50 years, as the carbohydrate increased, the percentage of calories from fat gradually decreased because of its known relationship to heart disease. It is important to note that currently, the percentage of carbohydrate is individually based on the dietitian's nutrition assessment and each individual's treatment goals.

Home blood glucose monitoring in the 1980s helped reveal how people with diabetes can eat a realistic amount of carbohydrate, based on factors such as blood glucose control, weight, and blood fat levels.

WHAT ARE STARCH AND FIBER?

As we learned in Chapter 2, starch and fiber are commonly known as *complex carbohydrates*. Starch and fiber are only found in plants, and their structure is composed of 10 or more straight or branched chains of sugar blocks called *polysaccharides*. Plants store their fuel as starch, so when we eat foods that come from plants, it is converted into glucose for fuel. Because starch is made up of many sugar blocks bonded together, these sugar blocks have to be broken down into their components before they can be used for fuel. The cooking, chewing, and digestive process breaks the bonds holding the sugar blocks together. A couple of hours after eating, all the starch is usually digested and is being used as fuel by the cells of the body.

The best sources of starch are grains, such as rice, wheat, corn, millet, rye, barley, and oats. Legumes (plants from the bean and pea family) and tubers such as potatoes and yams also provide starch.

WHAT IS FIBER?

Fiber is the "roughage" that comes from plant foods that cannot be digested by the human digestive system. It is considered the *non-starch polysaccharide* and is made up of cellulose, hemicellulose, pectins, gums, mucilages, and lignins. Fiber is what gives plants their structure and is found in all plant foods. Fiber is also the carbohydrate that gives bulk to the digestive tract. Unlike sugar and starch, fiber cannot give us fuel for energy because we cannot break the bonds that hold its sugar blocks together. Therefore, fiber only gives us very limited amounts of fuel and calories.

WHERE ARE STARCH AND FIBER FOUND?

Starch

A strong, healthful meal plan should feature foods rich in starch and fiber, such as breads, cereals, rice, pasta, dry beans, and starchy vegetables. The healthiest choices of breads and cereals are those made from whole grains, in which the whole kernel of grain is left in the flour used to make them. White flour has the bran (coarse outer layer) removed from the kernel of grain for a lighter texture.

Some specific foods in this category, commonly known as the Bread/Starch List, are listed below to give you an idea of how much one serving, or 15 grams of carbohydrate, would be:

Carbohydrate Foods: Breads, Cereals, Rice, Pasta, and Starchy Vegetables

Each of these items contains 15 grams of carbohydrate.
- 1 slice of whole-grain bread
- 1/2 English muffin or small bagel
- 3/4 cup dry cereal or 1/2 cup hot cereal
- 1/3 cup rice, beans, lentils
- 1/2 cup pasta, potato, corn, green peas
- 3 Tbsp flour
- 4–6 crackers
- 3 cups popcorn

Fiber

Fiber is categorized as either soluble or insoluble on the basis of its ability or inability to dissolve in water, respectively. Both soluble and insoluble fibers are called *dietary fiber*. This term is simply a measure of how much fiber is in a food.

Fiber that dissolves in water is called *soluble fiber* and includes such foods as citrus fruits, apples, strawberries, oat, wheat, rice bran, barley, leafy vegetables, and dried peas and beans. Soluble fiber cannot retain its structure in the digestion process and forms a gel that binds cholesterol and fats and helps to eliminate them from the body. Soluble fiber also slows the process of food emptying from the stomach. This can mean a slower rise in blood glucose levels after a meal containing adequate fiber.

Fiber that does not dissolve in water is called *insoluble fiber* and includes such foods as whole-grain cereals, wheat and corn bran, and mature fruits and vegetables, particularly root vegetables. Insoluble fiber works in the colon and has a sponge-like effect that helps push the food through the digestive tract.

WHY DO WE NEED STARCH AND FIBER?

All complex carbohydrates such as grains, breads, cereal, rice, pasta, fruits, vegetables, and legumes are healthy sources of fuel when eaten in moderation. Dessert-type foods that are high in sugar usually do not provide significant fiber, may contain a lot of fat, and are often limited in nutrition. Although sugar (a simple carbohydrate) is also a source of fuel, it should also be eaten in moderation. However, foods like fruits, vegetables, and milk contain forms of sugar as well as many other nutrients and are healthy sources of fuel. Some foods may contain both simple and complex carbohydrate. For example, fruits and vegetables contain both sugar and fiber. Most starches, as well as fruits, vegetables, and legumes, are low in fat and contain many nutrients, including fiber, vitamins, beta carotene, folic acid, zinc, iron, calcium, and selenium. The bulk of our diet, whether we have diabetes or not, should come from complex carbohydrates. They will keep us healthy!

Starch Is Used as a Fat Replacer

When fats are taken out of foods, the most common ingredient used to substitute the fat is a carbohydrate-based replacer in the form of a modified food starch. These food starches provide thickening and gelling abilities. They also stabilize, add texture, and provide structure to an otherwise unstable product. Common foods that may contain fat replacers are frozen desserts, baked goods, sauces, salad dressings, cheese, and gelatin. Often there is more than one fat replacer in the same food. You may recognize some of these carbohydrate-based fat replacers that come from corn, potato, rice, and tapioca, as well as ingredients such as polydextrose and maltodextrin. These fat replacers may cut down the amount of fat in a product but will raise the total carbohydrate content of these foods. It is very important to look at the grams of total carbohydrate on a food label when purchasing any low-fat or fat-free product because these products commonly contain more carbohydrate than expected. Remember that *carbohydrate* has the biggest impact on blood glucose.

Here's an example. Let's say you're looking at two bottles of blue cheese salad dressing—one is a light dressing and the other is a fat-free dressing.

	Light Blue Cheese Dressing	Fat-Free Blue Cheese Dressing
Serving Size	2 Tbsp	2 Tbsp
Total Fat	7 grams	0 grams
Total Carbohydrate	2 grams	11 grams
Fat Replacers	Tapioca, xanthan gum, modified food starch	Cellulose gel, maltodextrin, modified food starch, kayara gum

As you can see above, there's quite a bit of difference between the two dressings. This demonstrates the need to read food labels and monitor blood glucose after eating these foods to better understand how they will affect you.

The Upside and the Downside of Starch and Fiber

The good news for people with diabetes is that *all* carbohydrate foods can fit into a healthy diet, including starch or fiber. The body breaks down all carbohydrate, except fiber, into glucose (blood sugar) at the same rate, although this may be influenced by factors such as the presence of fat and protein in the same meal. Therefore, first and foremost, it is important to control the total amount of carbohydrate you eat.

The Downside

1. Eating a lot of carbohydrate from starch can lead to weight gain, even with the added benefits of vitamins, minerals, and fiber. Excess calories from any food will be stored as body fat.

2. Starchy foods, such as cake, cookies, muffins, sweet breads, and cereals, have higher amounts of total carbohydrate because of the starch plus the added sugar. Even though these foods may be part of a healthy diet, they may lead to higher blood glucose levels and weight gain. Therefore, the portion sizes should be carefully monitored.

3. If taken in excessive amounts, even fiber may be harmful. If a lot of fiber is consumed in a short period of time, it can cause intestinal gas, bloating, cramps, and constipation. Eating too much fiber, which absorbs water, can also lead to dehydration. When increasing fiber in your diet, do it gradually, giving your body time to adjust, and increase the amount of fluids you drink to at least 6–8 cups per day. Fiber in very large amounts can also interfere with the absorption of some minerals, such as zinc, iron, magnesium, and calcium.

The Upside

1. Whole-grain, high-fiber foods tend to be low in fat and calories (fiber does not provide calories or fuel) and can often prevent you from eating too much fat and protein from animal products. This

can reduce your risks of heart disease, overweight, constipation, and high blood glucose levels.

2. Whole-grain, high-fiber foods make us feel full and satisfied at meals and snacks without adding extra calories, and they help prevent overeating or going back for an extra helping. These foods also take longer to chew, so your brain has adequate time to notify your stomach that you are full.

3. Whole-grain, high-fiber foods form a large bulk in the intestine and help push the food through the digestive tract at a faster rate. This results in less pressure on the walls of the intestine, which reduces the risk of constipation, hemorrhoids, and diverticulosis.

4. Research has shown that by eating more soluble fiber, you can reduce risk of heart disease by lowering your LDL (bad) cholesterol.

HERE'S WHAT YOU CAN DO

1. **Get healthy.** A healthy fiber intake should be between 20 and 35 grams each day. This means that many Americans would have to double their intake.

2. **Variety can add fiber.** Eat a variety of carbohydrate foods to ensure that you get the health benefits from both soluble and insoluble fiber.

3. **Eat more vegetables.** Eat three or more servings of vegetables a day: 1 serving equals 1/2 cup cooked or 1 cup raw vegetables.

4. **Eat two or more servings of fruit each day.** One serving equals 1 small piece of fruit, 1/2 cup canned fruit, or 1 cup of cut-up fresh fruit.

5. **Eat at least six servings of grain products and legumes a day.** One serving equals 1 slice whole-

grain bread, 1/3 cup brown rice or pasta, 1 small potato with the skin, or 1/2 cup legumes or oatmeal. Tip: Add a handful of beans to a salad.

6. **Eat fewer processed foods.** Make sure the label's first ingredient on breads, cereals, and crackers is whole-grain flour, such as whole-wheat flour instead of just wheat flour or enriched wheat flour. Whole-wheat bread is not the same as wheat bread.

7. **Substitute items.** Use low-fat, low-calorie toppings (for example, 1 Tbsp salsa or 1 Tbsp nonfat sour cream) on starchy foods instead of the high-fat toppings, which add too many calories.

8. **Get more from your foods.** For extra fiber, leave the skin and peels on fruits and vegetables, if possible. Fruits with seeds, such as raspberries and strawberries, also contain a lot of fiber.

9. **Use whole-grain flours when cooking and baking.**

10. **Get help before taking supplements.** Check with your doctor or dietitian before taking a fiber pill or supplement. Fiber replacements lack other nutrients found in actual fiber-containing foods and often don't contain that much fiber anyway.

11. **Add a few sprinkles.** Sprinkle some ground flaxseed into your morning cereal or add it to your salad or yogurt.

SUMMARY

For years, starch has been thought of as the "fattening" ingredient in foods. Don't forget, however, that many starchy foods are eaten with added fat! When we eat potatoes, bread, corn, pasta, and vegetables, we rarely eat them without putting some sort of fat on them—butter, margarine, sour cream, cream cheese, and cheese sauce. What about a pasta meal? Not only are we served large quantities of pasta, but we also add several slices of Italian bread, breaded cutlets, and tomato sauce, with croutons on the salad, most of which contain carbohydrate in the form of starch. By the end of the meal, the carbohydrate has added up to an excessive amount. It isn't the starch or the pasta that causes weight gain and high blood glucose levels, it's the *total amount of calories from carbohydrate* and the *fat and protein* that was consumed.

Three nutrients provide fuel to the human body: carbohydrate, protein, and fat. Protein foods provide the most expensive fuel, take longer to empty from the stomach, and do not provide the quantity of fuel that carbohydrate does. Because Americans already eat too much protein and animal products, which puts us at a high risk for heart disease, many can not afford to add more, either financially or in terms of our health. Unfortunately, the brain and the central nervous system do not use the fuel from fatty foods efficiently. Fat also provides twice as many calories as carbohydrate and protein and is linked to insulin resistance, overweight, and obesity when consumed in large amounts. So that leaves us with carbohydrate, the major fuel source for our body. Food starch is probably the *most important* fuel source for energy and the *most preferred* fuel used by our brains and nervous system.

Contrary to what you hear from promoters of the many low-carbohydrate diets now on the market, low-carbohydrate diets dismiss evidence offered by well-known researchers and proven studies and condemn carbohydrate as the culprit in the development of diabetes, high blood sugars, and weight gain. The 2005 U.S. Department of Agriculture Dietary Guidelines actually directs Americans on how to eat in a balanced and healthy way by eating plenty of carbohydrate and fiber-rich foods, moderate amounts of protein, and low amounts of fat.

YOUR TURN

Now it's your turn to recall some key points from this chapter. Let's see how you do!

1. All Americans should be eating 20–35 grams of fiber per day, whether they have diabetes or not. True or false?

2. Fiber is only found in plant foods. True or false?

3. The fiber most helpful in lowering cholesterol and fats in the blood is _____ fiber.

4. The one type of carbohydrate that helps us feel "full" and satisfied after a meal is _____.

See APPENDIX A for the answers.

CHAPTER 4

PROTEIN

MYTH

People with diabetes should follow a high-protein diet to stay healthy and strong.

MARK: I've been reading that I should probably be on a high-protein, low-carbohydrate diet to help keep my blood sugars down.

DIETITIAN: While it is important to get enough protein in our diets to stay healthy, most of us get more than we need. We still need to get most of our calories from carbohydrate rather than protein, even if you have diabetes, because our bodies use carbohydrate for energy.

MARK: Okay, but because I'm exercising more to lose weight, plus lifting weights, shouldn't I be eating a lot of protein or even taking protein supplements to build more muscle?

DIETITIAN: Actually, the only way to really build stronger muscles is with regular exercise and a meal plan that contains anywhere from 40 to 60% of calories from carbohydrate, not from taking protein supplements or eating large portions of protein. Too much protein may even be harmful to your kidneys, especially if your doctor told you that you are spilling some protein in your urine.

WHAT'S NEXT?

Like Mark, most people think they don't get enough protein in their diets. There have been so many misconceptions over the years about protein and what it can do for us that we sometimes wonder if we truly get enough. Protein has practically been touted as a miracle nutrient. Several popular diets claim that eating more protein and less carbohydrate can help you melt away the pounds.

Many people with diabetes often end up eating more protein and less carbohydrate in an effort to control blood glucose levels. If you're looking to "bulk up," you may have tried protein powders that are often sold in health food stores (after all, muscles are made of protein, so it makes sense to eat more protein to build bigger muscles, right?). Yet, most of us eat too much protein, often at the expense of other nutrients, which can potentially lead to some serious health problems. Let's take a look at the truth behind some of these misconceptions about protein.

THE OLD AND THE NEW

The history of the role of protein in the diets of people with diabetes has been long and ever changing. Before the discovery of insulin, the only course of treatment involved dietary measures. Because people with diabetes were extremely limited in the amount of carbohydrate they could eat, the prescribed diets were usually high in protein and/or fat and often involved eating very strange foods, such as suet, blood, and even 10–40 egg yolks every day! Bread, pasta, and even fruit were off limits.

In the early 1900s, Dr. Elliot Joslin recommend limiting protein intake to 1 gram per kilogram of body weight because too much protein in the diet was found to increase both nitrogen and glucose in the urine, further aggravating diabetes. Have you ever been told that approximately 50–60% of the protein that you eat gets converted into blood sugar? This information came about in the 1930s using eggs, casein, and meat as the basis for studies of how protein affects metabolism in people with diabetes. Some health care professionals still use this information today, although more recent studies have challenged whether this "fact" is indeed true.

Much has changed over the years regarding the best diet for someone with diabetes. Because there are only three main nutrients to work with, diets have ranged from high fat to high protein to high carbohydrate. Even today, with some of the most advanced treatments for diabetes ever, leading health and diabetes authorities still can't agree upon the best diet for people with diabetes. Some believe a higher-protein diet is best, whereas others argue that a high-carbohydrate diet is the way to go, because a higher-protein diet could lead to some possible health problems down the road. Who is right? Although we may not have a definitive answer right now, read on to learn more about this controversial nutrient.

WHAT IS PROTEIN?

The word "protein" comes from the Greek word *proteios*, which means "of the first rank." No wonder we give it such importance in our diets! A protein is an organic substance made up of carbon, hydrogen, and oxygen (just like carbohydrate), but unlike carbohydrate, protein also contains nitrogen. These atoms are arranged into amino acids, which are linked into chains to form protein molecules. Amino acids are the building blocks of proteins, and there are 22 amino acids that are linked together in various combinations to form different types of protein molecules. Nine of these amino acids are called "essential" because our bodies cannot make them; they must be obtained from foods that we eat. It is important that we eat foods that contain essential amino acids because our cells need all 22 amino acids to make body proteins.

Why Do We Need Protein?

Protein has many important functions in the body. These include:

- creating new cells when old ones die
- forming antibodies (which fight viruses and bacteria)
- creating visual pigment to help us see
- forming enzymes (for example, digestive enzymes)
- forming certain hormones (such as insulin)

All of the cells in our bodies contain protein. In fact, approximately 50% of the body's weight comes from protein. Our hair, nails, muscle, cartilage, bone, and body fluids contain many different kinds of protein.

When we eat foods that contain protein, the protein is broken down into its building blocks, the amino acids. Our bodies then decide how those amino acids will be used and arrange the amino acids in a specific order, based on what types of proteins are needed. For example, the protein needed to help blood to clot (called thrombin) will have a different sequence of amino acids than the kind of protein needed to make insulin. Whatever amino acids are left over from protein synthesis will be stored as...you guessed right, fat.

How Much Protein Do We Need?

Most people in the U.S. grow up believing that a meal isn't a meal unless it contains a source of protein, usually in the form of a piece of steak, a hamburger, or a chicken breast. After all, who could stay healthy just by eating a plate of spaghetti? Surprisingly, although we do need to eat protein every day, we need much less than you may think. On average, people in the U.S. get approximately 15% of their calories from protein, which translates into 1.5 grams of protein per kilogram body weight. This is *twice* what is needed to meet our daily requirements, whether we have diabetes or not. Only about three percent of Americans have a protein intake that is below the recommended amount.

The recommended dietary allowance (RDA) for protein is 0.8 grams per kilogram body weight for adults. (We actually need only 0.6 grams of protein per kilogram body weight to stay healthy, but a margin of safety is built into the RDA). To give you an example, a man who weighs 170 pounds (77 kg) needs 62 grams of protein in his diet every day. A woman who weighs 130 pounds (59 kg) only needs 47 grams per day. Infants, children, and adolescents require more protein for growth and development; therefore the RDAs are higher (0.9–2.2 grams per kilogram of body weight per day). Protein needs are increased during pregnancy and lactation as well.

Diabetes and Protein Requirements

You've learned that there is no longer a set diabetic diet for people with diabetes. The best "diet" is one that will help you best control your diabetes and stay healthy. Also, recommendations for various nutrients can vary, depending on the type of diabetes you have and how well you are able to manage your diabetes. The American Diabetes Association states that there's no good evidence that aiming for a protein intake between 15 and 20% of calories should be modified.

More recently, however, some studies are showing that people with type 2 diabetes may actually *benefit* from a slightly higher protein intake. The theory that approximately 50–60% of protein in the diet gets converted to blood glucose (dating back to the early part of this century) has been challenged. A few studies have shown that blood glucose levels do not rise in people with type 2 diabetes who eat a diet containing a moderate amount of protein. Perhaps not as much protein is metabolized into glucose as we once thought. A similar effect has been seen in people with type 1 diabetes, although large amounts of protein do require more insulin to prevent high blood glucose levels (insulin is needed to help the body use protein, fat, and carbohydrate). Other studies have shown that a slightly higher intake of protein may lead to more weight loss compared with a more traditional, lower-fat eating plan and can even lower your risk for heart disease. Furthermore, eating a little more protein can help curb your appetite while preserving lean body mass if you're trying to lose weight. For these very reasons, the Joslin Diabetes Center nutrition guideline for people with type 2 diabetes recommends that between 20 and 30% of calories come from protein.

Does this mean that if you have type 2 diabetes you can eat more protein in your diet without it affecting your diabetes control? The answer varies from person to person. The best way for you to determine how protein affects *your* blood glucose control, whether for a meal or a snack, is to be diligent about checking your blood glucose levels after eating. It's also important not to eat too much protein because extra protein means extra calories. There is also the risk of too much protein worsening diabetic kidney disease and leading to other health problems, such as osteoporosis, kidney stones, and possibly certain types of cancer. It's important to talk with your dietitian about how much protein you need to stay healthy.

WHERE IS PROTEIN FOUND?

Once you know how much protein you need every day, you then need to learn what foods contain protein. However, you most likely know this already! Chances are, you are picturing steak, pork chops, turkey, and fish. *Animal sources* of protein include:
- red meats (beef, pork lamb, veal)
- poultry (chicken, turkey, duck, goose)
- seafood (fish, shellfish)
- dairy foods (milk, yogurt, cheese, eggs)

These animal protein foods contain all of the essential amino acids; therefore, they are often called "complete" protein foods. These foods provide adequate protein to meet the body's protein needs. It is relatively easy for both men and women to meet their daily protein requirements by eating fairly small amounts of protein.

Let's first calculate how much protein a 130-pound woman requires each day:

$$130 \text{ lbs} \div 2.2 = 59 \text{ kilograms (kg)}$$
$$59 \text{ kg} \times 0.8 \text{ g/kg} = 47 \text{ g protein per day}$$

We can then figure out how she can meet this daily requirement by eating animal sources of protein:

Example	Protein content
4 ounces tuna	28 grams
1/2 cup cottage cheese	14 grams
1 cup nonfat milk	8 grams
Total	**50 grams**

As you can see, this woman's daily protein needs can easily be met by eating just these three sources of animal protein. It is no more challenging for men to meet their protein needs, even though they need more than women, because men tend to eat more than women, anyway.

The main problem with animal protein is that you get more than you bargain for. Animal sources of protein are often high in fat, mainly saturated fat. Saturated fat, in turn, is responsible for raising cholesterol levels, which can lead to heart disease. Because the majority of our protein intake comes from animal sources, it's really no surprise that our fat intake has also increased. Some of these animal foods contain more calories from fat than from protein. It's important to make sure you choose the leanest forms of animal protein foods to avoid the dangers of excess fat in your diet, which include obesity, heart disease, and cancer.

Protein Content of Animal Foods

Food (4 ounces, cooked, unless noted)	Protein (grams)
Chicken breast, skinless	35
Turkey breast, skinless	33
Pork tenderloin, trimmed of fat	34
Beef, sirloin	34
Tuna, packed in water	28
Fish (cod, flounder, haddock)	21–30
Eggs, 2 large	14
Cottage cheese, 1% milkfat, 1/2 cup	14
Milk, nonfat, 1 cup	8

Protein from Plants?

Believe it or not, plants also contain protein, in addition to carbohydrate. In fact, someone who is a vegetarian probably gets most of his or her protein from plant foods. You may be curious (or even somewhat skeptical) about these plant proteins—just where *are* they found? A primary source of plant protein is from the *legumes*, or dried beans and peas. Examples are:

- kidney beans
- chickpeas (garbanzo beans)
- black beans
- soy beans
- lentils
- split peas

One-half cup of beans or peas contains 8 grams of protein, which is the amount of protein found in 1 ounce of meat, poultry, or fish. Keep in mind that this same serving of beans or peas also contains about 15 grams of carbohydrate.

Other sources of plant proteins are soy foods (tofu, soymilk, soy cheese, etc.), nuts, seeds, and "meat analogs," which are vegetarian-style (meatless) versions of typical meat foods, such as burgers, hot dogs, and sausage. Meat analogs are made from soybeans, vegetables, and/or grains, such as oatmeal. Remember that these foods eaten alone will not supply you with all of those essential amino acids we mentioned earlier. But you can get the amino acids by combining them with other foods. Are you turning up your nose at this point? Well, here are some very common foods that you probably already eat that are "complete" protein foods:

- peanut butter and jelly sandwiches
- black beans and rice
- vegetarian chili
- refried beans and tortilla chips
- minestrone soup
- hummus (chickpea spread) and pita bread

The beans or nuts and the grain foods (bread, rice, pasta, or tortillas) complement each other. When they are paired up, they provide you with protein just like that found in meat.

Why would you want to eat plant protein foods instead of animal protein foods? Well, for several reasons. First, plant-based meals tend to be healthier for you. You already know that many animal protein foods are high in both total fat and saturated fat. Plant protein foods are lower in fat, low in saturated fat, and contain more fiber. Second, plant-based meals add variety to your weekly menus. Third, meatless meals can be easy on your budget. Plant protein foods are much less expensive than meat, poultry, or fish.

THE UPSIDE AND THE DOWNSIDE OF PROTEIN

The Role of Protein in Diabetes and Kidney Disease

Diabetic kidney disease, called *nephropathy*, is one of the major complications of diabetes. The kidneys act like filters in the body, working to remove toxic substances. The substances that are removed are excreted in the urine. Uncontrolled diabetes can lead to damage of the small filtering units of the kidney called *glomeruli*. Normally, glomeruli work to keep certain particles, such as protein, from being expelled in the urine. If these glomeruli are damaged, which can sometimes happen with diabetes, protein molecules can slip through and enter the urine. A small amount of protein in the urine, called *microalbuminuria*, is an early sign of kidney damage.

We know how important protein is for staying healthy. But for people with kidney disease, sometimes eating large amounts of protein is too much of a good thing. In fact, a high-protein diet can be downright harmful. Although there are still some conflicting opinions about the role of protein in kidney disease, there are good studies showing that a lower-protein diet may actually prevent kidney disease from worsening. People with end-stage renal failure often feel much better if they follow a lower-protein diet because fewer nitrogenous wastes (wastes created when the body processes protein) build up in their blood.

Many physicians and dietitians recommend that people with diabetes who have early nephropathy start to cut back on their protein intake. Does this mean you should stop eating protein? Of course not. A lower-protein diet must be carefully planned, preferably by a dietitian, to make sure you don't eat *too little* protein. A lower-protein diet does mean, however, that you need to eat smaller portions of meat, poultry, and fish, as well as limit the amount of dairy foods, such as milk, cheese, yogurt, and eggs, that you eat. There is some evidence that eating more vegetable protein foods may be less harmful to the kidneys than eating animal protein foods. If you are following a lower-protein diet already and would like to try more plant-based meals, speak with your dietitian.

Too *Little* Protein?

So far, you've learned that people tend to eat too much protein and that too much protein may not be so healthy, especially for people with diabetes and kidney problems. What about not eating enough protein? Is this possible in a country known for thick steaks, fried chicken, and clambakes? Unfortunately, protein malnutrition is common in some Third World countries that are unable to adequately feed their citizens. However, the U.S. also has groups of people at risk for protein malnutrition, including low-income families, pregnant women who do not eat enough, alcoholics, and, at higher risk, older adults. Data from the National Health and Nutrition Examination Survey indicates that up to 25% of older Americans do not consume the RDA for protein. In fact, these people may be eating only half of the protein that they need.

An elderly person who lives on a diet of "tea and toast" may lose lean body mass, which is mostly muscle. This, in turn, can lead to loss of strength and decreased muscle contraction, putting that person at risk for falls and injury. Insufficient protein intake can also impair the immune system, making that person more susceptible to disease and lengthening the recovery time from an illness or surgery. Obviously, older people need to make sure they eat a variety of foods, including poultry, fish, lean meats, dairy products, and/or legumes to make sure that they get enough of this important nutrient.

Weight Loss and High-Protein Diets

High-protein, low-carbohydrate diets have been around for several decades. Remember Dr. Atkin's *Diet Revolution*? The Stillman Diet? The Scarsdale Diet? The Beverly Hills

Diet? In recent years a fresh batch of new diets—*The Zone, Dr. Atkin's New Diet Revolution,* and *The South Beach Diet*— have appeared, many of which tout the same claims as their older cousins. The underlying premise for most of these books is that a low-fat, high-carbohydrate diet can actually make you fat because carbohydrates cause the body to release insulin, which, in turn, leads to fat storage. What many readers who are desperate for the quick, easy solution to permanent weight loss do not realize is that there are no good studies showing that insulin causes weight gain (a common theme found in many of these books). Unfortunately, they may be led to believe that these lower-carbohydrate, higher-protein diets are the answer to their weight-loss woes, particularly when they actually do lose weight.

How can we explain the weight loss that does result from these diets? Well, what they have in common is that they all manage to cut calories, some more drastically than others. There really is no special magic here. Whenever you decrease your caloric intake, weight loss will result. Keep in mind, too, that some of these diets have much more fat, especially saturated fat, than we should be consuming, which may spell trouble for your arteries down the road. Plus, if you follow the advice of some of these diets, you'll find yourself following strict rules as to when you can eat, what you can eat, and what combinations of foods you can eat. Once again, there is no solid evidence backing up these claims. As we mentioned earlier, a slightly higher protein intake may help people lose weight—along the lines of 30% of calories from protein and no less than 130 grams of carbohydrate per day. But ultra-low carbohydrate plans are not realistic, or healthy, to follow for long periods of time.

Remember that, right now, there is no quick, super-easy way to shed those pounds. Eating right and exercising are still the key. What you choose to eat makes a big difference. Although health authorities may disagree on exact percentages, a good goal is to aim for roughly 50%

of your calories to come from carbohydrate, 15–20% from protein, and no more than 35% of calories from fat. So far, this seems to be the magic formula, especially when you eat whole-grain foods, fruits, vegetables, and lean protein foods. Oh, and don't forget to take that 30-minute walk!

HERE'S WHAT YOU CAN DO

1. **Calculate your own daily protein requirements.** As stated earlier, the RDA for protein is 0.8 grams of protein for every kilogram of body weight. If working with kilograms is confusing for you, use the table below to figure out how much protein you need every day. Keep in mind, too, that protein requirements are based on a healthy body weight, not necessarily how much you actually weigh. In other words, this doesn't mean that you need more protein if you are overweight. Multiply your *healthy* body weight by the number of grams of protein listed below to determine your daily protein requirements:

Adults 19 years and older	0.36
Pregnant women	0.62
Lactating women	0.53

   Your weight (in pounds) × number from above = daily protein requirement (in grams)

2. **Keep your portion sizes in check.** Men and women typically need no more than 3–6 ounces of protein each day. Three ounces is about the size of a deck of playing cards. So if your idea of a decent-size piece of steak is 12 ounces, which is more like four decks of cards, you might want to cut back a little.

3. **Choose lean sources of protein.** Lower-fat protein foods have no more than 3 grams of total fat per serving. Try lower-fat versions of cheeses and

processed meats. Aim to fit more plant-based protein foods into your meal plan.

4. **Eat at least one meatless meal per week.** How about trying vegetable lasagna, beans and rice, or soy burgers? Serve a grain food, such as brown rice or whole-grain couscous, as the main dish instead of as a side to chicken or hamburgers. Toss some tofu into your stir-fry or mix some vegetarian hamburger into your chili. Meatless meals don't have to be bland or boring!

5. **Talk to a dietitian.** A registered dietitian can help you learn how to best fit plant-based foods into your meal plan to make sure you're getting the proper nutrition, learn how to eat enough protein without getting too much fat, and learn how to balance your meal plan so that you're not eating more protein than your body needs. A dietitian will also help you determine how much protein you need, based on factors such as the type of diabetes you have, your weight, and your level of diabetes management.

6. **Don't fall for fad diets.** Tempting as they may be, talk to your health care provider before you buy into a high-protein, low-carbohydrate diet. These kinds of diets can be dangerous, especially if you have underlying kidney disease. If you want to lose weight, your dietitian can help you adjust your meal plan so you lose weight safely.

SUMMARY

In this chapter, you've learned that protein is an essential nutrient. Without it, we wouldn't survive. Protein is found in an abundant supply of foods such as poultry, seafood, meats, dairy foods, and even plant foods such as legumes (dried beans and peas). Most people in the U.S., with a few exceptions, eat enough protein. Too much protein, however, is not healthy, especially for people with diabetic kidney disease. Once again, by eating a variety of foods you can rest assured that you will get enough protein.

YOUR TURN

Now it's your turn to recall some key points from this chapter. Let's see how you do!

1. People with kidney disease should not eat any protein. True or false?

2. List three different animal protein foods:

    _____

    _____

    _____

3. List three different sources of plant protein foods:

    _____

    _____

    _____

4. Plan to eat one meatless meal during the upcoming week. Write down the meal you plan to try:

    _____

See APPENDIX A for the answers.

CHAPTER 5

FAT

MYTH

People with diabetes have to follow a rigid fat-free diet.

BRADY: The "diabetic diet" should be called the "NO" diet—no fat, no sugar, no fun! I had my annual checkup last week, and I brought in my laboratory results so that you can help me interpret them. The doctor told me to make an appointment with you right away because my "good" cholesterol is too low and my "bad" cholesterol and triglyceride levels are too high. I try to limit fried foods and eggs—what more can I do?

DIETITIAN: Our goal is to avoid diets that are completely fat free. Not only are they impossible to follow, but they will also leave you feeling hungry more often, which leads to more frequent snacking. The goal for most Americans, including those with diabetes, is to eat a moderate amount of fat. This means limiting "unhealthy" fats and including more "healthy" fats in their place. Because people with diabetes are at a higher risk of developing hardening or blockage of the arteries, heart disease, and stroke, it is very important that you know how the types and amounts of fat you eat play a role in increasing these health risks. That is why your doctor measures the levels of fat in your blood at your checkups.

BRADY: I travel constantly for my job and end up eating at the airport and in restaurants many weekdays. Needless to say, I regularly eat fast food, so I have also gained about 15 pounds over the past year. I guess I'll have to add no calories to my "NO" list!

DIETITIAN: Today, we are going to discuss eating in a heart-healthy way. The good news is that when you cut down on unhealthy fats and focus on moderate amounts of healthy fats, you will also get rid of a lot of calories in the process and still feel more satisfied after eating a meal. Fat contains more than twice as many calories as carbohydrate and protein. The same fat guidelines are no different than those suggested for everyone, with and without diabetes.

BRADY: Well, I guess it's about time I started concentrating on my health and taking the time to plan what and when I'm going to eat every day. I guess no more fast food.

DIETITIAN: You don't have to give up all your favorite foods. Everyone needs *some* fat for good health. Let's discuss how you can still fit in your favorite foods but limit how often you eat them.

WHAT'S NEXT?

Brady and his dietitian immediately developed a heart-healthy plan. Even though he was still often eating at the same restaurants, he was now making better, healthier food choices on his own. Instead of trying to eat "fat free," Brady learned that although all fats are high in calories and some are more unhealthy than others, he could limit how often and how much of these foods he ate and still keep his favorite foods as part of his overall healthy food intake. He was eventually able to lower his "bad" cholesterol and triglyceride levels and increase his "good" cholesterol level without medication.

THE OLD AND THE NEW

In the days before the discovery of insulin, people with diabetes were advised to get about 70% of their calories from fat every day. This was because fat is concentrated in calories and known to have the least effect on blood glucose levels. Fat was one nutrient that those with diabetes could eat to ensure adequate calories and still gain some control of their blood glucose. Common sources of fat in the so-called "diabetic diet" included lots of cream, butter, oil, lard, mayonnaise, whole milk, nuts, and bacon, along with eggs, cheese, and peanut butter.

The discovery of insulin, however, allowed people with diabetes to increase their intake of carbohydrate and therefore lower their fat intake. In 1950, the nutrition recommendation for fat intake dropped to about 40% of total daily calories, less than the pre-insulin days, but finally the start of a downward trend in fat intake. By 1971, the recommendation for fat dropped to 35% of calories, and again down to less than 30% in 1986. This decrease was due to research studies that linked fat to the number one cause of death in our country, heart disease. Research also showed that lowering blood cholesterol levels could lower chances of having problems with the heart and blood vessels.

Making dietary changes is the first approach to addressing high fat levels in the blood, before using cholesterol-lowering medications. Currently, the American Diabetes Association's nutrition recommendations state that the distribution of calories from fat and carbohydrate should be tailored to the individual person. The percentage of calories from fat depends on the individual's goals for blood glucose and fat levels, as well as for weight. People with normal blood fat levels who are at a desirable weight may be advised to have 35% or less of their total daily calories from fat. Those with abnormal blood fat levels and who are overweight may be advised to have 20–25% of their total daily calories from fat.

WHAT IS FAT?

Have you ever heard the term "blood lipids"? Lipid is simply another word for fats. Most of the fats in our food and in our body are called *triglycerides*. Another member of the lipid family is *cholesterol*. When we talk about cardiovascular disease or high cholesterol levels, we talk about cutting down on *dietary fat* (which includes triglycerides, saturated fat, trans-fat, and unsaturated fat) and *dietary cholesterol*, both of which come from the food we eat. When we talk about the blood test done at the doctor's office called a lipid profile, we are talking about blood fat (or triglycerides) and blood cholesterol (which includes total cholesterol and HDL and LDL cholesterol) or levels of these found in the blood. Basically, we are talking about fats in food and fats in the blood and, more specifically, how to change and decrease the fats in the food so we have less fat in the blood. So, when your doctor tells you that you have hyperlipidemia, it actually means that you have too much cholesterol and/or fat in your blood.

We often hear of fats categorized as "good" and "bad." What this is really referring to are the different forms of fats: saturated, monounsaturated, polyunsaturated, and trans-fats. Their level of saturation or solidness distinguishes these fats. This has to do with the chemical structure of fats and the solidity of the structure. A *saturated fat* is more solid at room temperature than an *unsaturated fat*, which tends to be softer or more liquid at room temperature. Research has shown that eating a lot of saturated and trans-fats causes blood cholesterol levels to rise, more so than eating a lot of foods that are high in cholesterol.

WHAT IS CHOLESTEROL?

Cholesterol is a fat-like, waxy substance that is found in our bodies and also in specific foods we eat. Probably the most important fact about cholesterol is that it is only found in animal foods. These animal foods may include meat, fish, poultry, eggs, and dairy products. Plant foods do not contain cholesterol. Besides getting cholesterol from animal foods, our body produces cholesterol; therefore, it is *not essential* in our diet. So, we get cholesterol in two ways: in the animal products we eat and produced by our liver in the body. Blood cholesterol comes mostly from fat in foods, particularly saturated and trans-fats.

Fat and cholesterol are traveling companions in the bloodstream. A protein carrier called a lipoprotein transports them through the bloodstream. Generally, you can think of a lipoprotein as a wagon carrying fat and cholesterol. Because blood is a water-based substance and fat is an oil-based substance, fat cannot mix with water or travel in the bloodstream without help. This means that fat and cholesterol must be carried through the blood in a protein particle (the wagon).

There are two major lipoproteins that your doctor measures and has probably mentioned: high-density lipoproteins (HDL) and low-density lipoproteins (LDL). The high-density lipoproteins (HDL), made by the liver, carry less cholesterol and fat but more protein. This means that HDL is high in density. It can carry the cholesterol away from the arteries and cells and back to the liver for recycling or elimination. The low-density

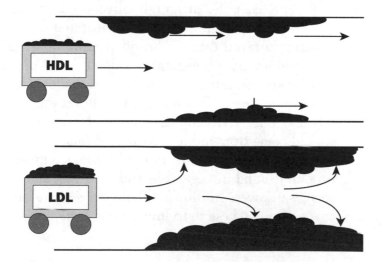

lipoproteins (LDL), also made by the liver, carry a lot of cholesterol and fat and less protein. This means that LDL is low in density. It can deposit cholesterol and fat on the artery walls and cells, causing a buildup in the body.

LDL is closely related to heart disease because high levels form the harmful fatty deposits that clog arteries and put you at a higher risk for heart attack and stroke. HDL seems to have a protective effect on the heart. If your HDL level is high, you are at a lower risk of heart disease. Remember, there is only one cholesterol. The HDL and LDL simply tell us the amount of fat and proteins being carried in them.

WHERE IS FAT FOUND?

We mentioned previously that fats are categorized according to their structure and level of saturation or "fullness." We also noted that the saturated (or solid) fats in the diet are the fats that cause blood cholesterol levels to rise. Now, let's talk about which fats are the most heart healthy and the most heart harmful to the body.

The most important thing to know about healthy and harmful fats is that they both contain the same amount of calories. So watching quantity as well as quality is essential if you want to lower your weight and cholesterol levels. Keep in mind that no fat or oil is made up of just one kind of fat. For example, although olive oil is mostly monounsaturated fat, about 20% of it is saturated fat.

> **Monounsaturated fats** are liquid at room temperature and found in vegetable oils such as olive, canola, and peanut oils as well as avocados, nuts, and olives. These help lower LDL cholesterol and possibly raise HDL cholesterol. Most of your fats should come from monounsaturated fats.

> **Polyunsaturated fats** are liquid at room temperature and found in vegetable and seed oils, such as corn, safflower, sunflower, flaxseed, sesame, and soybean oils. These help lower your LDL and pos-

sibly raise HDL. Polyunsaturated fats can be further classified into two categories:

- **Omega-6 polyunsaturated fats** are found in grains, nuts, and corn oil. Omega-6 fats help maintain healthy skin and body cells.

- **Omega-3 polyunsaturated fats** are found in canola, wheat germ, and soybean oil; flaxseed; nuts; and fatty fish. Omega-3 fats may help reduce the risk of heart attacks and strokes.

Saturated fats are solid at room temperature. These fats come mainly from animal sources and are found in butter, meat, lard, poultry skin, whole milk, cheese, sour cream, cream cheese, yogurt, and coconut, cocoa butter (chocolate), palm oil, and palm kernel oil. These are the culprits that raise cholesterol levels in the blood. They lower HDL and raise LDL.

Trans-fats are partially solid at room temperature. These are made from the polyunsaturated vegetable oils. Through a process called *hydrogenation*, liquid oil is changed into a solid or partially solid fat. Examples of foods that contain trans-fats include some margarines and shortenings, cakes, cookies, crackers, donuts, French fries, chips, and other baked goods. Trans-fats are very common because hydrogenating fats gives food a longer shelf life and a pleasant feel in the mouth. They do, however, raise your blood cholesterol levels like saturated fats and may actually be more harmful than saturated fats because they lower HDL and raise LDL levels and can also increase triglyceride levels.

A healthy eating plan that is low in saturated and trans-fats as well as cholesterol (less than 200 grams per day) is often the first line of defense in lowering LDL cholesterol and triglycerides. Your intake of these fats should be moderate and carefully monitored. Keep this in mind as a general guideline: the softer or more liquid the fat, the better.

WHY DO WE NEED FAT?

Fat is useful and is necessary for good health. Fat is our storage form of calories (or energy) and is accessible (mostly from the fat cells) if food is not available or if extra energy is needed for activity. Fats have more than twice as many calories as carbohydrate and protein and can store more than twice as many calories in a small space. For survival purposes, fat storage is beneficial because it serves as a concentrated source of energy, but too much storage and too little physical activity can be harmful when it leads to overweight or obesity.

A layer of fat under the skin insulates the body against extreme temperatures and also cushions the important organs. Fat also makes up the outer structure of body cells, like a protective barrier. For example, if your hands are in constant contact with strong soap and water, you can damage the fat layer in the skin cells, which eventually leaves the skin dry and cracked.

One of the most important functions of fat is to provide important nutrients, namely the fat-soluble vitamins A, D, E, and K. These fat-soluble vitamins are mainly found in foods that contain fat and can only be carried by fat through the blood to cells in the body. Finally, fat provides flavor, tenderness, aroma, and palatability to the foods we eat.

Cholesterol is produced in the liver and is essential for life. Cholesterol is used in the digestion of fats and is the main ingredient in many hormones. It helps form vitamin D and is an essential part of the membranes of every cell in the body.

THE UPSIDE AND THE DOWNSIDE OF FAT

Fat has received particularly bad press in recent years. Although many Americans need to cut down on their fat intake, some have become fat phobic. They are eating less than 20% of their total daily calories from fat, and to make up for the calories lost from fat, they end up eating too many calories, mostly from carbohydrate. So as our fat intake has decreased in the U.S. from 40% of our total daily calories to less than 33%, the total number of calories per person has risen 7%. Health experts are now thinking that eating too little fat isn't healthy and that maybe a little more fat should be added as long as it's coming from unsaturated fats, preferably monounsaturated fats.

The Downside

1. **Extra calories.** Fat has more than twice as many calories as carbohydrate and protein, so even small amounts can add up to extra pounds. There are nine calories in every gram of fat, compared with four calories in every gram of carbohydrate or protein.

2. **Clogged arteries.** If you eat too many saturated and trans-fats, your arteries can become clogged, eventually cutting off the blood supply to the heart, brain, legs, and feet.

3. **Chronic disease link.** A high-fat diet increases the risks of heart disease, obesity, high blood pressure, and possibly some types of cancer.

4. **Small portion sizes.** Fat carries so many calories that it has to be eaten in small portion sizes. For example, *one level teaspoon* of margarine, butter, all types of oils, and mayonnaise is *one full serving size* or *one full portion of fat*. A serving size of regular salad dressing is *one level tablespoon*. A light or nonfat version of salad dressing is a better choice if you are unable to stick to smaller portion sizes. Remember to check the carbohydrate content in these products!

5. **Fat-free is not calorie-free.** In low-fat and fatfree products, fat is usually replaced with carbohydrate. Therefore, the total number of calories is

often not reduced, and if eaten in large amounts, these products can still raise blood glucose.

The Upside

1. **Fat is a useful food additive.** Fat provides flavor, enhances taste, adds moistness, acts as a tenderizer and preservative, and contributes to the creamy, crunchy, and crispy feel of foods. It is also responsible for the wonderful smells of certain foods.

2. **Fat storage has unlimited capacity.** Stored body fat provides the energy you need during exercise or long periods of food deprivation.

3. **Fat provides protection for the body.** Body fat keeps the body warm and protects it against shock and injury.

4. **Fat is a carrier of certain vitamins.** Fat provides vitamins A, D, E, and K.

HERE'S WHAT YOU CAN DO

1. **Get a lipid profile.** Ask your doctor for a lipid profile on a yearly basis or more often if you have hyperlipidemia. A lipid profile is a laboratory blood test that requires a small blood sample. This profile tells you what your blood levels are for total cholesterol, LDL cholesterol, HDL cholesterol, and triglycerides. Compare your results with the following recommended levels:

HDL cholesterol:	more than 40 mg/dl for women more than 50 mg/dl for men
LDL cholesterol:	100 mg/dl or less less than 70 mg/dl for those with diabetes and heart disease
Triglycerides:	less than 150 mg/dl

2. **Make an appointment with a registered dietitian.** A dietitian can help you determine how much fat you should be eating each day. This is different for all people and depends on many factors, such as weight, age, activity level, cultural background, total calorie intake, lipid levels, and family history of heart disease.

3. **Investigate your risk factors for heart disease.** Those risk factors that are either controllable or have a relationship with food intake are in italics.

Major Risk Factors for Heart Disease

Age: Over 45 years for men

Over 54 years for women

Women with premature menopause and
    no estrogen replacement therapy

Family history of premature heart disease

Cigarette smoking

*High blood pressure (over 140/90 mmHg or taking high
blood pressure medication)*

Low HDL cholesterol (less than 35 mg/dl)

High LDL cholesterol (greater than 130 mg/dl)

Low physical activity level

Obesity

Diabetes

---

4. **Practice moderation.** No foods have to be cut completely out of your diet. You may just have to eat some foods less often and in smaller amounts.

5. **Substitute unsaturated fats for saturated fats.** Use more low-fat or "light" products when having salad dressing, mayonnaise, cream cheese, sour cream, and milk.

6. **Instead of frying, try to broil, steam, bake, or grill your foods.**

7. **Remove the skin from poultry and trim the fat off meat.**

8. **Use only half the amount of oil in recipes and in main dishes.** If you do use oil, use monounsaturated oil, such as olive, canola, or peanut oil, or purchase these in nonstick cooking sprays.

9. **Read food labels.** The upper part of the food label will tell you how many calories come from fat. As long as your daily intake of fat is 20–35% of your total calories, it is okay if an individual food is higher. Total Fat grams per serving and how much of the Total Fat is coming from Saturated Fat or Trans-Fat are listed just below the Calories. Some manufacturers might even tell you the amount of monounsaturated and polyunsaturated fats. Also, look at the nutrient claims for fat and remember that the fat claims only apply to *one serving*.

SUMMARY

Taking control of your health by decreasing your intake of unhealthy fats, and therefore decreasing your risk of heart disease, is an important goal. Lowering your health risks requires regular visits with your diabetes team. Your team will help inform you about healthy eating. Make a list of your risk factors for heart disease and work to address those factors that you do have some control over, such as cigarette smoking and physical activity level. Also, focus on those risk factors that are controllable and have a relationship with food, such as obesity, high blood pressure, diabetes, low HDL cholesterol, and high LDL cholesterol. Research has shown that by replacing saturated and trans-fats with monounsaturated and polyunsaturated fats, you can greatly lower your risk of heart disease.

Your best bet is to be realistic and flexible. Make small changes over time and balance your food choices over the course of a day. Remember that although the quality of the food is important, you should be sensible and focus on the quantity of food you are eating.

YOUR TURN

Now it's your turn to recall some key points from this chapter. Let's see how you do!

1. Cholesterol comes only from animal sources and our liver. True or false?

2. A _____ fat is more solid at room temperature than an unsaturated fat, which is liquid at room temperature.

3. High-density lipoproteins are considered healthy because they are carrying more protein and less _____.

4. Low-density lipoproteins are considered less healthy because they are carrying less _____ and more fat.

5. Which of the following statements refer to the positive roles that fat plays?

   _____ protects our major organs

   _____ provides lots of calories

   _____ helps lower cholesterol levels

   _____ stores vitamins A, D, E, and K

   _____ prevents dry skin

   _____ intensifies the taste of foods

   _____ maintains our body temperature

   _____ provides fiber

See APPENDIX A for the answers.

CHAPTER 6

SUGAR SUBSTITUTES

MYTH

People with diabetes should only eat sugar-free foods.

SANDY: I am trying to be good and only buy sugar-free foods, but I've noticed that my blood glucose sometimes goes up after I eat some sugar-free foods and that I frequently have stomach aches. What does this all mean?

DIETITIAN: You might be surprised to learn that "sugar free" does not necessarily mean calorie free or carbohydrate free and that some sugar substitutes may not have a significant benefit over regular sugars.

SANDY: Do you mean that I can't eat unlimited amounts of sugar-free food?

DIETITIAN: It is important to know that there are two types of sugar substitutes: those that *do not* provide calories and carbohydrate and those that *do* provide calories and carbohydrate, which can affect your blood glucose and even your weight! What this means is that many foods with sugar substitutes must be counted into your eating plan. Furthermore, when eaten in large quantities, some of these caloric sugar substitutes may have a laxative effect because they are not well absorbed in your digestive tract.

SANDY: Well, if I still have to count some of these sugar substitutes as part of my carbohydrate allowance, couldn't I use my carbohydrate allowance on *regular* foods?

DIETITIAN: Absolutely—the choice is yours. Within the context of a healthy diet, you can spend your carbohydrate allowance on any food you choose.

WHAT'S NEXT

Sandy was very surprised to learn that non-nutritive (no-calorie) sweeteners (aspartame, saccharin, acesulfame potassium, sucralose, and neotame) offer the advantage of allowing people with diabetes to enjoy the sweet taste that most of us desire in foods without negatively affecting blood glucose and weight. However, the nutritive (calorie-containing) sweeteners (the sugar alcohols, fructose, polydextrose, and maltodextrin) do provide both calories and carbohydrate. Sandy was taught that some sugar substitutes, such as the sugar alcohols, may produce a slightly lower rise in blood glucose because they are poorly absorbed in the digestive tract and therefore provide fewer calories. However, they must still be counted as part of her carbohydrate allowance in her eating plan. The American Diabetes Association nutrition recommendations state that calorie-containing nutritive sweeteners may not be significantly healthier than foods sweetened with regular sugars in regard to reducing the intake of calories and carbohydrate or improving blood glucose levels.

THE OLD AND THE NEW

So-called "diabetic foods" began emerging over 100 years ago, due to the numerous and often unattainable restrictions of the "diabetic diet." Because people with diabetes enjoyed the same sweet properties of foods as much as those without diabetes, sugar substitutes became a necessity.

For the past 40 years, due to the thinking that all sugar should be avoided in the diabetic diet because of its perceived rapid absorption and resulting rise in blood glucose, sugar substitutes became common ingredients added to a wide variety of foods. The adaptation of special "diabetic" products seemed to expand the quality of life for people with diabetes. After all, these products *did* help people with diabetes follow a healthier eating plan. Many of these foods were also used for weight control by those without diabetes.

Today, with our knowledge of sugar and its effects on blood glucose, we know that if sweetness is needed, using sugar alcohols, high-intensity sweeteners, and/or regular sugars (such as sucrose and fructose) are all acceptable. However, because some sugar substitutes contain calories, they are not necessarily beneficial for weight loss or blood glucose control. Many people with diabetes wrongly assume that foods containing sugar substitutes can be eaten as "free foods." This assumption often has a negative effect on blood glucose levels and weight management. Just like any other food, those containing sugar substitutes have to be accounted for in an eating plan.

Before 1970, our food goals were mostly focused on food safety and nutritional deficiencies. Today, our goals have changed focus and evaluate how food relates to healthy living and disease prevention. Because of our plentiful food supply and the resulting overweight and obesity issues in our country, the perceived need for low-calorie foods is in high demand. Let's take a look at the facts, so if you do choose to use sugar substitutes, you will be able to manage your blood glucose and weight.

HERE ARE THE FACTS

Sweeteners fall into one of two categories: non-nutritive or nutritive. These categories separate sweeteners into those without calories (non-nutritive) and those with calories (nutritive). Other terms used to describe these sweeteners are *sugar substitutes*, *sugar replacers*, or *alternative sweeteners*.

Non-Nutritive: High-Intensity Sweeteners

Currently five high-intensity sweeteners are regulated for food use: saccharin, aspartame, acesulfame-K, sucralose, and neotame. All high-intensity sweeteners are identified as food additives; provide a lot of sweetness in small amounts; offer sweet taste without calories, carbohydrate, or response from blood glucose; and do not promote tooth decay. The current trend is to blend different high-intensity sweeteners so that less sweetener is needed to obtain a sweeter, improved taste. So, a blend might include aspartame and acesulfame-K and still not provide calories.

Because high-intensity sweeteners are food additives, they must be assigned a safety limit, which is known as the Acceptable Daily Intake (ADI). The ADI is the estimated amount of sweetener, based on body weight, that a person can safely consume every day over a lifetime without risk. The ADI is a conservative amount and provides a 100-fold safety factor.

Saccharin

Saccharin is 200–700 times sweeter than table sugar (sucrose). It is heat stable and can be used in cooking. It is not broken down by the body and is eliminated. It is used as a tabletop sweetener (Sweet 'n' Low) and in chewing gum, cosmetics, medications, foods, and beverages. The ADI is 5 milligrams per kilogram of body weight per day. One packet of tabletop saccharin contains 40 milligrams.

Aspartame

Aspartame, better known as NutraSweet or Equal, has 4 calories per gram, but because it can be used in such small quantities, the amount of calories it adds to a product is negligible. It is 160–220 times sweeter than table sugar.

Aspartame is not heat stable and may lose some of its sweetness after long exposure to high temperatures. It is rapidly broken down in the digestive tract and does not build up in the body at recommended intakes. It is used as a tabletop sweetener and in carbonated beverages, powdered drinks, yogurt, gelatin, cereals, and frozen desserts. The ADI is 50 milligrams per kilogram of body weight per day. One packet of tabletop aspartame contains 37 milligrams.

Acesulfame-K

Acesulfame-K (or acesulfame potassium) is better known under the brand name Sunette and has no calories. It is 200 times sweeter than table sugar. Acesulfame-K is heat stable and can be used in cooking. It not broken down by the body and is eliminated. It is used as a tabletop sweetener and as an additive in chewing gum, confections, desserts, yogurt, sauces, and alcoholic beverages. The ADI of acesulfame-K is 15 milligrams per kilogram of body weight per day. A packet of tabletop acesulfame-K contains 50 milligrams.

Sucralose

Sucralose, better known under the brand name Splenda, has no calories and is 600 times sweeter than table sugar. It is heat stable and can be used in cooking. It is not broken down by the body and is eliminated. It is used as a tabletop sweetener and in desserts, confections, and non-alcoholic drinks. The ADI is 5–15 milligrams per kilogram of body weight per day. A packet of tabletop sucralose contains 5 milligrams.

Neotame

Neotame has no calories and is 7,000–13,000 times sweeter than table sugar. It is heat stable and can be used in cooking. It is used as a sweetener in breakfast cereals, processed fruits, frozen desserts, toppings, toothpaste, and beverages. The ADI is 2 milligrams per kilogram of body weight per day. A 12-oz beverage contains about 6 milligrams of neotame.

Nutritive Sweeteners: Sugar Alcohols

Experts agree that you can eat foods with sugar as long as you work them into your eating plan, just as you would with any other carbohydrate-containing food. This applies to nutritive sweeteners as well. Foods labeled as "sugar-free," "no sugar added," "reduced sugar," and "dietetic" still contain carbohydrate. Keep in mind that the Nutrition Facts label will list both added sugars and naturally occurring sugars (under grams of Total Carbohydrate), such as the natural sugar in milk (lactose).

The nutritive sweeteners include sugar, fructose, corn syrup, and many others described in Chapter 2. Also in the same category of nutritive sweeteners are the sugar alcohols, maltodextrin, and polydextrose. Although the U.S. Food and Drug Administration (FDA) defines high-intensity non-nutritive sweeteners as food additives, the FDA considers nutritive sweeteners like the sugar alcohols as Generally Recognized as Safe (GRAS) ingredients. The sugar alcohols most commonly found in foods are sorbitol, mannitol, xylitol, isomalt, and hydrogenated starch hydrolysates (HSH). Sugar alcohols come from plant products such as fruits and berries and are considered carbohydrates. These sugar substitutes can replace sugar sweeteners with somewhat fewer calories, producing a smaller rise in blood glucose. They can also decrease the risk of tooth decay. The sugar alcohols are absorbed more slowly and incompletely, often producing a laxative effect if eaten in excess.

Unfortunately, people with diabetes often do eat too many foods containing sugar alcohols, thinking of them as "free foods," like the high-intensity sweeteners. If this is the case, the sugar alcohols may contribute excessive calories and cause a rise in blood glucose. So, even though sugar alcohols are considered reduced-calorie sweeteners (they provide about half the calories of regular sugar), if their serving size is not followed and the calories and carbohydrate content are not accounted for in the eating plan, they may provide no significant benefit over regular sugars, like sucrose and fructose.

Although sugar alcohols are not completely absorbed and thus provide fewer calories, large amounts may actually lead to malabsorption, which can cause gas, cramping, bloating, or diarrhea. This is why products that contain a lot of sorbitol and mannitol have a label with this warning: "Excess consumption may have a laxative effect."

Know Your Nutritive Sugar Alcohols

- Sorbitol is used in candies, chewing gum, jams, jellies, baked goods, and frozen confections. It provides 2.6 calories per gram and is 50–70% as sweet as table sugar.
- Mannitol is used as a dusting agent for chewing gum and as a bulking agent in powdered foods. It provides 1.6 calories per grams and is 50–70% as sweet as table sugar.
- Xylitol is used in chewing gums, candies, pharmaceuticals, and oral hygiene products. It provides 2.4 calories per gram and is as sweet as sugar.
- Erythritol is used as a flavor enhancer and bulking agent and adds texture to foods. It provides 0.2 calories per gram. It is 60–80% as sweet as table sugar.
- Isomalt is used in confections and/or as a bulking agent. It provides 2 calories per gram and is 45–65% as sweet as table sugar.
- Maltitol is used in confections and/or as a bulking agent. It provides 2.1 calories per gram and is 90% as sweet as table sugar.
- Hydrogenated starch hydrolysates (HSH, or maltitol syrup) are used in confections and/or as bulking agents. They provide 3 calories per gram and are 24–50% as sweet as table sugar.

Blended Sweeteners

Sugar substitutes, both nutritive and non-nutritive, are often blended together. Sugar alcohols are usually less sweet than table sugar but add bulk to products, much like "regular" sugars. High-intensity sweeteners provide a concentrated sweetness in a very small volume but no bulk. Therefore, a blend could include a mixture of several sugar alcohols and a high-intensity sweetener. So if you see aspartame (non-nutritive) listed on the front of a package, you still have to look at the carbohydrate content on the food label to see if any sugar alcohols (nutritive) are blended with the aspartame. Remember that this blending does not constitute a free food.

HERE'S WHAT YOU CAN DO

Because we now know that not all sugar-free foods are created equal, the very first step when considering a sugar-free food is to check the food label. Below is a quick and easy way to find out if a high-intensity sweetener is the only sweetener in the product or if there is a blend of sugar alcohols with the high-intensity sweetener.

1. **Follow this quick guideline.** To avoid being misled, take the following steps. Look immediately at the Total Carbohydrate in one Serving Size on the Nutrition Facts label. If a Serving Size has 5 or fewer grams of Total Carbohydrate and has fewer than 25 calories, then it is counted as a free food. *You can stop right here.* Free foods should still be limited to no more than three or four servings spread out over the day.

2. **Cut back.** An option is to choose the regular version of a food and cut back on the serving size instead of buying the sugar-free version, which may also cost more (and may not taste as good, either).

3. **Count it if you have to.** If the food has a Total Carbohydrate content greater than 5 grams per serving size, then the carbohydrate amount has to count as part of your carbohydrate allowance.

4. **Carbohydrate has the biggest impact on your blood glucose.** You need to focus on the carbohydrate amount in a serving. However, if you focus on sugar (listed under Total Carbohydrate), you might be misled because you will likely see zero grams. Sugar alcohols do not have to be listed next to sugar (they are sugar substitutes), unless the term "sugar free" or "no added sugar" is used on the label. However, sugar alcohols and any sugar always have to be totaled in the grams of Total Carbohydrate. You will never be misled if you focus on the grams of Total Carbohydrate. The table on p. 82 illustrates this difference when choosing between sugar-free foods.

COMMONLY ASKED QUESTIONS

Are the sugar alcohols listed next to Sugars on the Nutrition Facts label?

Sugar alcohols are not listed on the food label next to Sugars or combined with the grams of sugar because they are sugar substitutes. However, if the manufacturer uses the term "sugar free" or "no added sugar" on the food label, the grams of sugar alcohols must be listed. If more than one sugar alcohol is in a product, the amount of sugar alcohol will be listed under the grams of Total Carbohydrate. If just one sugar alcohol is used in a product, its specific name (for example, sorbitol) is listed. However, sugar alcohols are always counted into the grams of Total Carbohydrate and must be accounted for in your eating plan. You will be misled if you only look at Sugars. The rule of thumb is that if there are 10 or more grams of sugar alcohol listed on the

Comparison of Sugar-Free Foods

Type of Food	Free Food	Sugar-Free Foods with Carbohydrate	
	Sugar-Free Gelatin	Sugar-Free Instant Pudding	Sugar-Free Hard Candy
Serving Size	1/4 package or 1/2 cup	1/4 package or 1/2 cup	4 pieces
Total Carbohydrate	0 grams	6 grams	15 grams
Sugars	0 grams	0 grams	0 grams
Sugar Substitutes	maltodextrin, aspartame, acesulfame-K	modified food starch, maltodextrin (from corn), aspartame, acesulfame-K	isomalt, acesulfame-K (Excess consumption may have a laxative effect)
One Serving	1/2 cup = free	1/2 cup = 1/2 carbohydrate serving or 1/2 slice of bread	4 pieces = 1 carbohydrate serving or 1 slice of bread

food label, then you can subtract *one-half* of the grams of Sugar Alcohols from the Total Carbohydrate grams because sugar alcohols are often poorly absorbed.

Does "no sugar added" mean the same thing as "sugar free"?

No, the terms have different meanings. "Sugar free" means that a food contains less than 0.5 grams of regular sugar per serving. This does not apply to sugar substitutes. "No sugar added" means that the processing and packing does not increase the sugar content over the amount *naturally* found in the ingredients. For example, a fat-free fruit yogurt made with aspartame may claim that it has "no sugar added" because it is sweetened with a sugar substitute in place of regular sucrose. However, it cannot be called "sugar free" because the product still contains sugar—the milk it is made with contains the natural sugar lactose and the fruit in it contains the natural sugar fructose.

I use sugar-free candy to treat hypoglycemia. Is this okay?

No, it is not recommended that you use these foods as treatment foods for hypoglycemia because they are more slowly absorbed from the digestive tract and may not work quickly enough to raise blood glucose levels. Also, many of these foods have a lot of fat per serving. Fat slows down stomach emptying and also does not work fast enough to raise your blood glucose.

YOUR TURN

Now it is your turn to recall some key points from this chapter. Let's see how you do!

1. All sweets that contain sugar substitutes have less fat and calories than the sugar-sweetened versions they are replacing. True or false?

2. Eating "no added sugar" or "sugar-free" foods may

raise your blood glucose and your weight. True or false?

3. Looking only at grams of Sugars on a food label may lead you to mistakenly believe that a food will not affect your blood glucose levels or your weight. True or false?

4. Which of the non-nutritive sweeteners is not heat stable and may lose its sweet taste after long exposure to high temperatures? _____

See APPENDIX A for the answers.

CHAPTER 7

CARBOHYDRATE COUNTING AND THE GLYCEMIC INDEX

MYTH

People with diabetes *must* follow a diabetic diet that uses exchanges (or choices) to plan their meals.

MARIA: I was diagnosed with diabetes over 15 years ago and have tried to follow a "diabetic exchange/choice diet" many times over the years, but in all honesty, I am embarrassed to admit that I have never fully understood how this diet works and neither have I ever been able to really stick with it. So, I just gave up! How do other people with diabetes do it? I guess I'm just a "bad" diabetic.

DIETITIAN: Don't be so hard on yourself, Maria. No one is perfect. Your main goal as a person living with diabetes is to maintain near-normal blood sugar levels by balancing your food intake with your diabetes medications and activity levels. My main goal as your dietitian is to help you make small, realistic changes in your eating that will improve your nutrition and blood sugar levels without totally altering your lifestyle.

MARIA: But, I've seen several dietitians over the years, and many seem so inflexible and judgmental. What's different now? I live with my mother, and she's a retired nurse. She told me about *carb counting* and the *glycemic index*. She said that I should be using these newer methods for better blood sugar and weight control. What are they?

DIETITIAN: You will be happy to know that dietitians are now able to offer more flexible guidelines rather than predetermined plans. Because nutrition is such an essential part of successful diabetes care—and often the most challenging part—health professionals have come to realize that one diet does not fit all people. Medical nutrition therapy requires an individualized approach that is appropriate for your personal lifestyle and cultural background. Carbohydrate counting is just a simple a way to keep track of how many carbohydrate foods you are eating at each meal and snack. It works kind of like an allowance. The glycemic index ranks these carbohydrate foods according to how much they may raise your blood sugar. Many people find these meal planning approaches easier to follow, and they allow you to fit in any food you like, as long as your overall eating is healthy.

MARIA: Do you mean I don't have to give up all of my favorite family foods and feel deprived and hungry all the time?

DIETITIAN: That's right! You and I will work together to develop a meal planning option that you are able and willing to do, and, most important, it will be realistic for your lifestyle.

WHAT'S NEXT

Those like Maria, who have had diabetes for many years, will never forget the many restrictions placed on them and their food choices when they were first diagnosed. Often they were made to feel that they lacked willpower or were just plain "cheating" when they were unable to stick to a rigid diet.

Because of the many changes that have taken place in the diabetes and nutrition field, we now know that there is no one diabetic or American Diabetes Association diet. Research has provided nutrition professionals with the opportunity to offer flexible guidelines rather than an artificial distribution of foods and/or rigid rules. Unfortunately, like Maria, many people with diabetes are unaware of these positive changes and new approaches. This dietitian was particularly happy to learn that Maria's mother was a primary support person and that her mother also wanted to learn the most up-to-date nutrition methods with Maria.

The first issue addressed by the dietitian was Maria's hunger and feelings of deprivation. Because Maria was a young, active woman in her thirties, the dietitian wanted to assess Maria's calorie needs and ensure that Maria received an adequate amount of calories every day. The dietitian explained that another important goal of nutrition therapy is to ensure that the person consumes adequate calories to maintain or attain a reasonable weight. Next, the dietitian asked Maria about her favorite foods, her usual food intake, her work week and weekend schedules, and overall activity level. Knowing this information ensured that the dietitian created an eating plan that distributed Maria's calories and carbohydrate allowance in a realistic way.

Maria and the dietitian discussed how diabetes, food, and activity interact and which meal planning option would best meet Maria's lifestyle. They both agreed that *carbohydrate counting* (and using the *glycemic index* as an additional tool) would be the most realistic option for Maria's lifestyle and the one best suited to help Maria meet her nutrition goals. Maria's renewed interest in diabetes self-management eventually allowed her to learn how to interpret her blood glucose numbers and to use this information when planning her meals and snacks.

THE OLD AND THE NEW

When anyone mentions diabetes and food choices, most people think of "strict, rigid diets," "hunger," "deprivation," "rules," "artificial or bland food," "no sugar," "lists of good and bad foods," and "taking the pleasure out of eating."

Even after the initiation of insulin therapy in 1921 and into 1950, there were no available standardized food lists that specified portion sizes for individual foods. Doctors and patients had to spend hours calculating, measuring, and strictly determining how much, when, and what the patient could eat. Food choices were rigid and monotonous, eating outside of the home was impossible, and casseroles or mixed dishes were rarely included.

Eventually, in 1950, the American Dietetic Association, the American Diabetes Association, and the U.S. Public Health Service devised a food exchange/choice system. This was simply a framework that grouped foods together that were similar in calories, carbohydrate, protein, and fat per serving. This system allowed foods from the same group to be substituted for each other and was to be universally used so that everyone would be using one uniform method to account for what they ate. This framework still exists today.

From this new method came preprinted tear-off sheets of standardized diets, which meant that health professionals did not have to spend time calculating individual diabetes diets. Unfortunately, these "diet sheets" did not take into account each individual person's likes or dislikes, cultural background, or overall lifestyle. When people with diabetes were unable to adhere to these "diet sheets," they were thought to be noncompliant, unmotivated, and difficult.

This exchange/choice system has continued to be updated and modified over the years while still maintaining the basic framework developed in 1950. The American Diabetes Association determined that choosing an appropriate meal planning method based on each person's ability, willingness, education level, and nutritional needs was necessary for the person to understand how to plan his or her meals. Because of the many differences in people with diabetes and their dietary needs, there had to be other available meal planning options to help people reach their healthy eating goals.

HERE ARE THE FACTS

There are seven meal-planning options currently in use today. Like Maria, many people with diabetes are curious to learn more about *carbohydrate counting* and the *glycemic index*. This counting approach has evolved to meet the demands of the person who wants to take charge of his or her diabetes self-management. Those people who use *only diet and exercise* or *diabetes pills* to control their diabetes can use these approaches to help monitor weight and blood sugars by regulating how much carbohydrate they eat at each meal and snack. Those on *insulin* may also use this approach to coordinate food intake, exercise, and insulin use by matching peak insulin activity with the peak levels of blood glucose that result from the digestion and absorption of carbohydrate foods. The glycemic index can then be incorporated as an additional tool to help on those days when blood glucose levels rise higher than expected.

The Diabetes Control and Complications Trial (DCCT) was a very large, multi-center diabetes study that began in the 1980s. The DCCT studied about 15,000 people with type 1 diabetes for a period of nearly 10 years. This study was able to demonstrate that *any* improvement in blood glucose management makes a difference in delaying the onset and progression of diabetes complications. Carbohydrate counting was used as one of the four meal planning approaches in the DCCT, and both patients and health professionals found that this system allowed more flexibility in food choices and helped them meet their diabetes self-management goals. Although carbohydrate counting has been around for many years, many people still think that the diabetic diet is based solely on the exchange/choice system.

Simply stated, carbohydrate counting is a meal planning approach that primarily focuses on the total amount of carbohydrate. This is based on the premise that almost 100% of the total carbohydrate from a meal is converted to blood sugar within the first few hours after eating. So you can see how eating a set amount of carbohydrate at each meal will keep your blood glucose level more consistent. This chart demonstrates why we focus on carbohydrate:

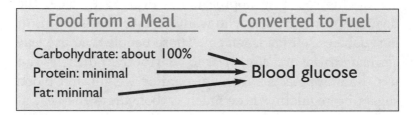

Food from a Meal	Converted to Fuel
Carbohydrate: about 100%	Blood glucose
Protein: minimal	
Fat: minimal	

All foods contain nutrients that have varying effects on blood sugars; however, only minimal amounts of the protein and fat are converted directly into blood sugar. This does not mean that we can simply ignore protein and fat. These nutrients may still affect blood glucose by slowing the stomach emptying process and by delaying the absorption of carbohydrate foods. Regardless of meal planning methods, healthy eating is always the main goal.

Exchanges/Choices Versus Carbohydrate Counting

Look at the chart on p. 91 to see how exchanges/choices can be converted to carbohydrate grams for carbohydrate counting.

You will note that instead of the six *separate* food groups under the exchange list/food choice system, the revised exchanges/choices simply groups the carbohydrate

Exchanges/Choices	Carbohydrate Counting
1 Starch/Bread	15 grams of carbohydrate
1 Fruit	15 grams of carbohydrate
1 Milk	15 grams of carbohydrate
1 Vegetable	0–5 grams of carbohydrate
1 Meat	no carbohydrate in protein
1 Fat	no carbohydrate in fat

foods together under one heading: the carbohydrate group. This incorporates the Starch/Bread, Fruit, Milk, Vegetable, and Other Carbohydrates exchanges into one group.

In other words, one serving of Starch/Bread, Fruit, and Milk all contain 15 grams of carbohydrate, which is equal to one carbohydrate choice:

$$\frac{1 \text{ Fruit Choice}}{15 \text{ grams of carb}} = \frac{1 \text{ Bread/Starch Choice}}{15 \text{ grams of carb}} = \frac{1 \text{ Milk Choice}}{15 \text{ grams of carb}}$$

Budgeting Your Carbohydrate Allowance

Every person needs a certain amount of fuel from food each day. The bulk of this fuel should come from healthy carbohydrate foods, although protein and fat contribute some. The carbohydrate foods make up our total carbohydrate budget. Think of the amount of carbohydrate as your daily allowance. Your carbohydrate allowance is like a budget and must be spread out between meals and snacks.

You should note that some foods contain more carbohydrate than other foods, such as cereals, candy, desserts, and sodas. Think of these foods as being more expensive foods, because they require you to spend a large amount of your carbohydrate allowance when you choose or buy them. Take a look at the following example.

> **You could choose to eat:**
> - 1/4 cup of maple syrup, which has about 50 grams of carbohydrate.
>
> **Or you could eat:**
> - 3 pancakes, which also has about 50 grams of carbohydrate.

The maple syrup may taste good, but the pancakes will fill you up and supply more nutrients to your body. How would you rather spend your 50 grams of carbohydrate? The main goal of carbohydrate counting is to wisely budget your carbohydrate allowance and get the most value from what you choose.

Glycemic Index

Now that you have learned the basic concept of carbohydrate counting, you can still make further improvements if you choose. The glycemic index is a system that rates foods by how fast they raise blood sugar levels. Foods are then ranked on a scale from 0 to 100. The higher the glycemic index number, the faster that particular food is digested and absorbed, thus raising blood sugar levels.

Generally, foods with a glycemic index less than 55 are called *low glycemic index foods* and those with a glycemic index higher than 70 are called *high glycemic index foods*. The glycemic index demonstrates that the impact of a food on your blood sugar level is determined not only by its sugar content, but also by how quickly it is digested and absorbed. In fact, many starchy foods are more rapidly absorbed than foods that are high in sugar. A diet that uses low glycemic index foods, is low in saturated and trans-fats, and is high in dietary fiber can lead to a healthier you.

Putting the Glycemic Index to Work

You do not have to be a math whiz to improve your glycemic control with the glycemic index. If you are using the glycemic index to help improve your blood sugar levels, the goal is to balance high and low glycemic index foods.

You may be thinking, "But can't I just eat only foods with a low glycemic index and avoid all foods with a high glycemic index?" Unfortunately, using the glycemic index is not as simple as that. Take a look at the chart below. It shows some high and low glycemic index foods. Notice that there are healthy and unhealthy foods on both lists. A healthy high glycemic index food, such as a baked potato with skin (without toppings), can provide important nutrients and fiber, whereas an unhealthy low glycemic index food, such as French fries, can cause weight gain. Remember, the glycemic index does not rate a food based on its vitamins, minerals, protein, fat, fiber, or calories, so you won't be able to create a nutritious meal plan based solely on the glycemic index. Other factors can also affect the glycemic index of a food.

High Glycemic Index Foods (more than 70)	Low Glycemic Index Foods (less than 55)
Cornflakes (84)	Apple (41)
Pretzels/Rice Cakes (81)	Banana (53)
Frozen Waffles (76)	Grapes (43)
Bagel (72)	Green Beans (less than 15)
Instant Rice (91)	Long-Grain Rice (47)
Cream of Wheat, Instant (74)	Old-Fashioned Oatmeal (not instant) (49)
Dates (103)	Fresh Orange Juice (52)
Bread, White (71)	Peach (28)
Doughnut, Cake Type (76)	Spaghetti (41)
Scones (92)	Sweet Potato (54)
Baked Potato (75)	Tomatoes (15)

- **Length of cooking time and processing.** Cooking and processing breaks down fiber and swells starches, which results in faster absorption and a high glycemic index.
- **The amount of fiber.** Tight, compact clumps of fiber are harder to digest, which means that a high-fiber food will have a low glycemic index.
- **The amount of fat.** The more fat in a food, the slower the carbohydrate is digested and absorbed, which means that it will have a low glycemic index.
- **The ripeness of fruits and vegetables.** Glycemic index increases as fruits and vegetables ripen.
- **The combination of foods served in a meal.** Combining foods will lower the meal's overall glycemic index.
- **The acid content of foods.** Vinegar and lemon slow the rate of digestion, which means that foods with high acidity have a low glycemic index.

HERE'S WHAT YOU CAN DO

We now know that the type and amount of food you eat, especially carbohydrate foods, determines how high and how fast your blood sugar level goes up. It is very important to know how many grams of carbohydrate you will be eating at each meal and snack, so you can foresee changes in blood sugar levels. Many people with diabetes feel that carbohydrate counting (paired with use of the glycemic index) is a more precise way to manage eating than by following exchanges/choices. Here are some tips to help you get in the fast lane to successful carbohydrate counting.

1. **Health professionals can help you.** Set up a visit with a registered dietitian (RD) who is also a certified diabetes educator (CDE) (Appendix B). This health care professional will work with you to determine your daily food requirements based

on your age, height, weight, and activity level, while taking into consideration your favorite foods, cultural background, and lifestyle. There is no set amount of carbohydrate that is recommended for all people with diabetes.

2. **Learn your carbohydrate budget and allowance.** The dietitian will help you add up the total number of grams of carbohydrate for each meal and snack and effectively spread out your carbohydrate to help you learn how to budget your carbohydrate allowance.

3. **Learn your portion sizes.** For a couple of weeks, practice learning portion sizes by measuring and weighing your food at meals. Eating too much carbohydrate at one time will raise your blood sugar, even if the food is healthy.

4. **Think about your appetite.** How much food will be needed to fill you up at each meal or snack? If you have budgeted 15–20 grams of carbohydrate for your bedtime snack, what would be more satisfying: 1/2 cup of ice cream (sugar free or not, it has about 15–20 grams of carbohydrate), 4–6 whole-grain crackers, or a small to medium orange? The carbohydrate cost for all of these is the same!

5. **Go from high to low glycemic index foods.** Change part of your daily carbohydrate intake from high glycemic index foods to low glycemic index foods or replace one high glycemic index food with one low glycemic index food per meal (for example, beans for potatoes, oatmeal for cornflakes).

6. **Lower the glycemic index of your favorite foods.** Avoid giving up a favorite food by lowering its glycemic index by adding fiber or a healthy fat. For instance, if you want to continue eating your favorite flake cereal, add a small handful of slivered almonds (healthy fat and fiber) to slow its absorption rate.

7. **Have a handy reference for carbohydrate counting.** Purchase a carbohydrate counting reference book at any bookstore or go to the American Diabetes Association website at http://store.diabetes.org. Reference books are helpful when you are eating a food that doesn't come with a Nutrition Facts label, as is the case with many of the meals we eat in restaurants.

8. **Have a handy reference for the glycemic index.** If you want to learn more about the glycemic index, purchase a glycemic index reference book or go to www.glycemicindex.com.

COMMONLY ASKED QUESTIONS

What about protein and fat? Aren't they important anymore?

The amounts of protein and fat that people eat are very important, and dietitians want to help people meet the recommended guidelines for healthy eating. Protein and fat are not our main focus when we count carbohydrates and neither do they affect the blood sugars as much as carbohydrate. However, if a dietitian notices that a person is adding high amounts of fat to his or her meals and snacks, the dietitian may work with the person to assign a certain number of fat servings to each day. If weight loss is needed or decreasing high cholesterol is a major goal, this will be taken into consideration. In addition, many Americans eat more protein per day than the amount actually needed by the body. Therefore, most people are given a guideline that translates their protein intake into a certain amount of ounces per day.

Is it best to eat only low glycemic index foods at every meal to see a benefit?

The effect of a low glycemic index food carries over to the next meal. However, why not aim for at least one low glycemic index food per meal? Remember to purchase more unprocessed foods that contain more fiber and slow the absorption of carbohydrate. Combining both high glycemic index and low glycemic index foods in a meal lowers the overall glycemic index of the entire meal.

What about animal products such as chicken, eggs, fish, meat, cheese, and nuts? Why are they not mentioned in the glycemic index lists?

These foods do not contain carbohydrate and will not have much of an impact on your blood glucose levels. Remember that the glycemic index is a ranking of carbohydrate foods.

Why not just eliminate all carbohydrate foods to keep my blood glucose levels from rising?

Eliminating carbohydrate from your diet is restrictive and not recommended. Carbohydrate is a very important nutrient and our main source of fuel and fiber. The National Academy of Sciences Food and Nutrition Board recommends that everyone eat at least 130 grams of carbohydrate per day to maintain proper brain and nervous system function.

YOUR TURN

Now it's your turn to recall some key points from this chapter. Let's see how you do!

1. You can only use carbohydrate counting if you are taking insulin. True or false?
2. When the body digests carbohydrate foods, almost ____ percent is converted into blood sugar. Only _____ amounts of protein and fat contribute to blood sugar.
3. Only low glycemic index foods should be eaten at meals and snacks. High glycemic index foods should be completely eliminated. True or false?

4. The amount of carbohydrate you should eat in a day is determined by a registered dietitian and you, based on your age, weight, activity level, and overall diabetes control. True or false?

See APPENDIX A for the answers.

CHAPTER 8

LABEL READING

> ## MYTH
>
> People with diabetes need to only look at sugar and calories on food labels.

RYAN: I got a call from my doctor's office last week after my yearly checkup. He told me that my cholesterol was high and that I needed to start eating better. He reminded me that I had gained about 15 pounds since my last visit before prescribing a new medication and increasing my insulin dose. I just spent over two hours at the grocery store trying to find foods to help me lose weight and lower my cholesterol level. Food labels have so much information! What should I be looking for when I look at food labels? I heard that if sugar or fat is listed in the first five ingredients, the food should be avoided.

DIETITIAN: You are not the only one who is confused about what to focus on when reading a food label. Although most people look at food labels, it is hard to understand what the numbers actually mean. With some education, you will be able to successfully read these labels.

RYAN: What about when a label claims that the product is fat free? Is it really fat free? What are net carbs?

DIETITIAN: I can show you a quick and easy way to look at food labels and help you interpret the most meaningful information for weight, cholesterol, and blood sugar management. By learning what items to focus on when reading a food label, you will be able to use your new knowledge to help you meet your particular needs.

RYAN: I brought some food labels with me today because these are some of the foods I eat often. I hope you can go over these with me.

DIETITIAN: Good idea. It is not necessary to give up your favorite foods as long as you know how to fit them into your meals or snacks. Let's get started.

WHAT'S NEXT

Food labels are supposed to provide us with easy-to-use nutrition information, yet many people have been known to spend hours at the grocery store trying to make sense of them. With some nutrition education, Ryan was amazed to learn just how quick and easy it was to read a food label and pick the foods that would help him meet his particular goals for weight loss, lowering cholesterol, and managing blood glucose. Now, when he walks down the grocery store aisles and sees hundreds of attractively packaged food items loaded with health claims, he no longer feels overwhelmed and restricted. He knows that a grocery list for a person with diabetes can contain a wide selection of healthy, tasty, and nutritious foods and includes the same foods that any healthy eater may buy.

THE OLD AND THE NEW

Nutrition labeling originally began in 1974 as a voluntary process for most foods. Labels were only required for products that added extra nutrients or made nutrition claims. Beginning in 1994, food manufacturers had to update their food labels when the federal government began regulating food labels. During the 1980s, food labels were confusing and untruthful and manufacturers were making meaningless health claims on their packaged foods. The Nutrition Labeling and Education Act of 1990 required food labels to display the following information.

Nutrition Facts

The information on the Nutrition Facts label is regulated and trustworthy. The label varies with every food product and contains product-specific information.

Serving Size

First, look at the serving size and the number of servings contained in the package. Ask yourself, "How many servings am I going to eat?" The nutrition information on labels is always for only a single serving. Serving sizes are standardized to make it easier to compare similar foods from one brand to another. Manufacturers used to make their serving sizes very small to make their foods seem lower in calories, fat, and sodium and to suggest that there were more servings in every container. The serving size on the label is now required to be a realistic amount that is represented in a format that people will easily understand, such as using "cups," "chips," or "pieces." However, if you have more than one serving of the indicated size, the nutrients on the label will need to be adjusted to match the number of servings that you are eating.

Calories

The number of servings you eat (your portion size) controls the number of calories you eat and how much energy (calories) you get from a serving of this food. In general, a food that provides 40 calories is low in calories, 100 calories is moderate, and 400 calories or more is high.

Nutrients

Americans usually eat sufficient or very large quantities of all five nutrients listed in the top half of the food label: Total Fat, Cholesterol, Sodium, Total Carbohydrate, and

Protein. The amount of the nutrients is expressed in two ways: the amount by weight per serving and as a percentage of the Daily Value, which is a nutrition reference tool. It is recommended that you include all five of these nutrients in moderation as part of a healthy, balanced diet.

Percent Daily Values

These values are listed on the right side of the label and help you to decide how much of a certain nutrient the food contributes without doing any calculations. If the food has a high percentage, it means that a serving goes a long way toward helping you meet your daily nutrition requirements. Remember, though, that these percentages are based on a daily 2,000-calorie diet.

Vitamins and Minerals

Food labels were originally designed to provide more information about vitamins and minerals in the latter part of the 20th century because Americans weren't getting all of the vitamins and minerals that they needed. Because few Americans are now deficient in the three B vitamins (thiamine, riboflavin, and niacin), they were removed from food labels. However, these and others may be added if *health claims* on the label mention their presence in the product. Currently, dietary fiber, vitamins A and C, and the minerals calcium and iron are listed because most Americans do not get enough of these.

Daily Values

The list of daily values is found at the bottom of the label and tells you how much of each kind of nutrient to eat each day. More specifically, the daily values indicate the amount that you use up when you eat one serving of that food. Although you may need more or less than the values listed, you can see what one serving of the food uses up.

Ingredients

The ingredients are listed in descending order of weight. The sources of some of the ingredients, such as flavorings, must be identified by name in case they need to be avoided for health or religious reasons.

HERE ARE THE FACTS

Health Claims

Due to widespread fraud and potentially harmful health claims on food labels in the 1970s and 1980s, health claims that link specific foods with lowering the risks of certain diseases are now strictly regulated. The Food and Drug Administration developed a policy that allows manufacturers to make only health claims that can be supported by scientific evidence. There are nine, and they are listed below.

1. Increased calcium intake can lower your risk of osteoporosis (loss of bone mass)
2. Reduced sodium intake can lower your risk of hypertension (high blood pressure)
3. Reduced dietary fat intake can reduce your risk of cancer
4. Reduced levels of saturated fat, trans-fat, and cholesterol intake can reduce the risk of coronary heart disease
5. Eating more fruits and vegetables can decrease the risk of cancer
6. Eating fruits, vegetables, and grain products that contain fiber (particularly soluble fiber) can decrease the risk of coronary heart disease
7. Eating fiber-containing grain products, fruits, and vegetables can decrease the risk of cancer
8. Adequate folate can lower the risk of neural tube defects during pregnancy
9. Dietary sugar alcohols do not cause dental caries (cavities)

Nutrient Content Claims

The food labeling regulations also set strict definitions to address the problem of misleading nutrition claims. When you see a term like "low fat," you can now believe it. The following nutrition terms are strictly regulated to describe a food's nutrient content.

Free

Other words may be used instead of "free," such as "without," "trivial or negligible source of," "no," "zero," or "insignificant source." Because it is impossible to measure below a certain amount of any nutrient, such as fat, when a food label claims that a product is "fat free," it actually means that there is less than one-half gram (0.5 grams) of fat per serving. Besides fat, "free" may also apply to cholesterol, sodium, sugars, and calories.

Low and Very Low

Other words may be used in place of "low," such as "little," "low source of," and "contains a small amount of." "Low" means that a person can eat a large amount of the food without exceeding the Daily Value for the nutrient. "Low" may describe total fat, saturated fat, cholesterol, sodium, and calories. The term "very low" can only describe sodium.

Fewer, Less, and More

These terms are used when a regular product is compared with a nutritionally altered product. The comparison food must be identified, and although the foods may not be exactly similar, they do have to fall within the same category. For example, a manufacturer can compare plain popcorn and potato chips. These are both snack foods, yet plain popcorn has 30% "less" or "fewer" calories than potato chips. In order to use the "more" claim, the food must have at least 10% more of the Daily Value for a particular nutrient than the reference food, for example, whole-wheat crackers have 10% more fiber than wheat crackers.

Light and Reduced

To use "light," "lite," or "reduced," the food must be comparable with a similar product within the same category and provide 25% less than what is in the original version, as in "light" ice cream compared with "regular" ice cream or "reduced-fat" cheese compared with "regular" cheese.

Lean and Extra Lean

These terms can only be used to describe the fat content of meat, poultry, seafood, and game meats. "Lean" foods are those with less than 10 grams of fat, less than 4 grams of saturated fat, and less than 95 milligrams of cholesterol per serving (about 3 oz) and may include chicken without the skin. "Extra lean" means the food has less than 5 grams of fat, less than 2 grams of saturated fat, and less than 95 milligrams of cholesterol per serving (3–4 oz) and may include fish, such as cod or haddock.

High and Good Source

In addition to "high," both "rich in" and "excellent source" can be used on products. The actual definition for "high" means that the food must have 20% or more of the Daily Value for that nutrient in a serving, whereas "good source" means that the food must have 10–19% of the Daily Value.

Common Terminology

Reading a food label can help you maintain and improve your health and your blood glucose control and weight, but only if you use it. In order to make the best food choices, you must be able to define the health claims and interpret the specific claims commonly used to describe specific nutrients. Here is a list of claims with which you should be familiar.

Calorie free: less than 5 calories per serving

Low calorie: 40 calories or less per serving

Reduced calories: at least 25% fewer calories per serving than that of the reference food

Sugar free: less than 0.5 gram of sugar per serving

No sugar added: processing and packing does not increase the sugar content over the amount naturally found in the ingredients

Reduced sugar: 25% less sugar per serving than in the reference food

Fat free: less than 0.5 gram of fat per serving

Saturated/trans-fat free: less than 0.5 gram per serving

Low saturated/trans-fat: 1 gram or less per serving

Low fat: 3 grams or less per serving

Reduced/less fat or saturated/trans-fat: 25% less per serving than that of the reference food

Cholesterol free: less than 2 milligrams of cholesterol or 2 grams or less of saturated fat per serving

Low cholesterol: 20 milligrams or less of cholesterol and 2 grams or less of saturated fat per serving

Reduced or less cholesterol: at least 25% less cholesterol and 2 grams or less of saturated fat per serving than that of the reference food

High fiber: 5 grams or more per serving and must also be low fat

Good source of fiber: 2.5–4.9 grams of fiber per serving

Added fiber: 2.5 grams or more of fiber per serving than in the reference food

Sodium free: less than 5 milligrams per serving

Very low sodium: 35 milligrams or less per serving

Low sodium: 140 milligrams or less per serving

Reduced sodium: at least 25% less sodium per serving than in the reference food

Net Impact Carbs

There are label controversies about carbohydrate-related terms, such as "Low Carb" and "Net Impact Carbs," that *are not* approved label claims. These products claim that blood glucose is not affected by certain carbs, and food companies have created their own terminology to add more marketing appeal to their products. Net impact carbs result from replacing wheat flour with soy flour or by adding sugar alcohols, fiber, or fat. These foods do contain carbohydrates and can affect blood glucose levels because they use sugar alcohols and contain carbohydrate (see Chapter 6) and fiber (see Chapter 3). These sugar alcohols can cause digestive problems because they are not absorbed and digested in the same way that sugar is. Keep in mind that "low carb" doesn't always mean "low calorie" and some of these products may contain more fat and calories than products that are not labeled as "low carb." So, if you want to eat lower-carbohydrate foods, read the Nutrition Facts label before you purchase your food. Turn to natural low-carbohydrate food sources, such as nuts, seeds, fruits, vegetables, whole grains, and healthy oils.

How to Read a Nutrition Facts Label

Let's start by thinking of *all* foods as being a possible choice for an eating plan, rather than putting foods into "good" or "bad" categories. Let's also think about a quick and easy way to look at any food label—regardless of which aisle you are standing in—without spending countless hours at the grocery store.

Simply looking at a bunch of numbers does not turn into useful nutrition knowledge. So ask yourself, "How will a serving of this particular food affect my blood sugars and my weight?" To do this, it is helpful to have some reference foods that you can easily visualize for comparison, so you can interpret what you are eating in terms of familiar food items. The following guidelines are quick, simple, and useful and can help you accurately interpret any food label.

Look at the Nutrition Facts label for a whole-grain cereal on p. 108. We'll go through this label step by step.

Check the Serving Size

When reading the Nutrition Facts label, always start at the top of the label so you won't miss anything. Remember that the serving size does not necessarily match the standardized portion sizes found in *Choose Your Foods: Exchange Lists for Diabetes*. Also, you have to seriously consider how much you will actually eat compared to the listed serving size. If you eat more than the stated serving size, you will need to adjust all of the nutrient numbers accordingly. If the serving size looks ridiculously small—for example, one cookie—you will have to ask yourself if you can eat only one serving and avoid having more. In cases such as these, it may be better if you leave this product on the shelf at the grocery store and do not bring it into your home. In the label on this page, the actual serving size is 1 cup (the 53 grams listed next to the serving size is the weight of each level cup of cereal).

Whole Grain Cereal

Nutrition Facts

Serving Size 1 cup (53g/1.9 oz)
Servings Per Container About 8

Amount Per Serving

Calories 190	**Calories from Fat** 25

	% Daily Value**
Total Fat 3g*	**5%**
Saturated Fat 0g	**0%**
Trans Fat 0g	
Cholesterol 0mg	**0%**
Sodium 95mg	**4%**
Potassium 300mg	**9%**
Total Carbohydrate 36g	**12%**
Dietary Fiber 8g	**32%**
Soluble Fiber 3g	
Sugars 13g	
Protein 9g	**14%**

Vitamin A 0%	•	Vitamin C 0%
Calcium 4%	•	Iron 10%
Phosphorus 10%	•	Magnesium 10%
Copper 8%		

*Amount in Cereal. One half cup of fat free milk contributes an additional 40 calories, 65mg sodium, 6g total carbohydrates (6g sugars), and 4g protein.
**Percent Daily Values are based on a 2,000 calorie diet. Your Daily Values may be higher or lower depending on your calorie needs.

	Calories:	2,000	2,500
Total Fat	Less than	65g	80g
Sat Fat	Less than	20g	25g
Cholesterol	Less than	300mg	300mg
Sodium	Less than	2,400mg	2,400mg
Potassium		3,500mg	3,500mg
Total Carbohydrate		300g	375g
Dietary Fiber		25g	30g

Calories per gram:
Fat 9 • Carbohydrate 4 • Protein 4

INGREDIENTS: Soy Grits, Hard Red Winter Wheat, Long Grain Brown Rice, Whole Grain Oats, Barley, Rye, Buckwheat, Sesame Seeds, Evaporated Cane Juice Syrup, Corn Meal, Corn Flour, Soy Protein, Wheat Bran, Oat Flour, Corn Bran, Honey, Natural Flavors, Calcium Carbonate, Salt

CONTAINS SOYBEAN AND WHEAT INGREDIENTS

Check the Total Fat

Working your way down from Serving Size, you'll notice that the food has a Total Fat of 3 grams. To decrease our risks of heart disease, cancer, and overweight, this category will immediately tell you if this particular food is a good choice. Remember that the 3 grams of Total Fat is the amount found in 1 level cup. If you glance below, you can see how much of the Total Fat comes from saturated or trans-fats. In this case, the whole-grain cereal meets the criteria for low total fat and no saturated or trans-fats.

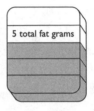

a pat of butter

What does 3 grams of fat look like? To easily visualize grams of fat, think of those pats of butter that you receive at restaurants (the ones stuck to cardboard and a slip of paper). Each little square of butter is 1 teaspoon of butter. A pat of butter is an example of one serving of fat, and one serving of fat always has 5 grams of fat. So, we will use a pat of butter as our reference food to indicate what one serving of fat looks like. Think of the pat of butter (1 tsp) being divided into five parts (5 grams). If you color in three of the parts (3 grams of fat), you can see how much fat is in each cup of whole-grain cereal. Because cereal typically does not contain fat, you can see in the ingredient list that the fat comes from the sesame seeds that have been added for flavor and fiber.

Check the Total Carbohydrate

For a quick and easy label check, we are now down to our last entry: Total Carbohydrate. When you read the Nutrition Facts label, you will see that 1 cup of this cereal has 36 grams of Total Carbohydrate and a total of 8 grams of Fiber. Fiber (see Chapter 3) may be deducted from the grams of Total Carbohydrate because it has little impact on blood glucose and contains very few calories. So 1 cup of cereal contains 28 grams of Total Carbohydrate (36 − 8 = 28) that needs to be counted. If this product had contained more than 10 grams of sugar alcohol, which is not completely digested, half of the grams could also be subtracted from the Total Carbohydrate.

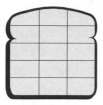

**a slice of bread
(15 total carb grams)**

What exactly does 28 grams of carbohydrate look like? To easily visualize grams of carbohydrate, think of a slice of bread. One slice of bread is an example of 1 carbohydrate (starch/bread) serving and is also easy for most people to visualize. One carbohydrate serving is equal to 15 grams of carbohydrate. Because all servings of carbohydrate foods do not have exactly 15 grams of carbohydrate, we can go up or down by 4 points, so 11–19 grams of carbohydrate is still the same as one carbohydrate serving. Think of a slice of bread being divided into 15 parts or having about 15 grams of carbohydrate. Each part is about one gram of carbohydrate.

Review

Let's review the information we have collected from this Nutrition Facts label.

- One level cup of whole-grain cereal has 3 grams of fat, which is a bit more than half of a pat of butter.
- One level cup of whole-grain cereal has 28 grams of carbohydrate, which is about two slices of whole-grain bread.

So, one level cup of whole-grain cereal will have the same effect on your blood glucose as if you had eaten two slices of whole-grain bread with a little more than half a pat of butter.

HERE'S WHAT YOU CAN DO

1. **Meet with an expert.** If you do not have an individualized meal plan or carbohydrate allowance, set up a meeting with a dietitian to determine the number of grams of carbohydrate, fiber, and fat you should aim for at each meal and snack.

2. **What is the bottom line for each food?** Every time you read a label, any label, ask yourself the following question: "If I eat one serving of this food, how many pats of butter and slices of bread will the food be equivalent to?" Here's another example. Which of these fits best into your eating plan?

	Nonfat Fruited Yogurt with Aspartame	Nonfat Fruited Yogurt without Aspartame
Serving size	8 ounces	8 ounces
Total fat	0 grams	0 grams
Total carbohydrate	18 grams	42 grams
Equivalent in bread	1 slice of bread	almost 3 slices of bread
Equivalent in pats of butter	0 pats of butter	0 pats of butter

3. **Read, read, and read more.** You will find out that you have been eliminating many foods that can easily fit into your meal plan. You will also begin to understand what caused some of those high blood glucose readings or extra pounds. For example, if you eat a whole deli bagel, you're actually taking in about 75 grams of carbohydrate. This is about the same as eating five slices of bread! Keep in mind that this doesn't include cream cheese, which adds extra fat to the meal as well.

4. **Read the Serving Size entries very carefully.** Foods like peanut butter are fine when eaten according to the serving size, but can be very high in fat and calories when portions are not moderated. Also, always verify information carefully—you can easily see that there is no difference in the

two peanut butters below, even though one claims "No Added Sugar." In cases like this, it is more important to stick with the listed serving sizes.

	Creamy Peanut Butter (Regular)	Creamy Peanut Butter (No Added Sugar)
Serving size	2 Tbsp (level)	2 Tbsp (level)
Total fat	17 grams	18 grams
Total carbohydrate	5 grams	6 grams
Equivalent in bread	1/3 slice of bread	1/3 slice of bread
Equivalent in pats of butter	3 1/2 pats of butter	3 1/2 pats of butter

5. **Compare No Sugar Added products with regular products.** You will notice that the carbohydrate content is often very similar between these two products. If you choose to spend your carbohydrate on the regular product instead of the no-sugar-added product, and the fat content is pretty much equal in both, then you can choose either product. Look at the ice creams below:

	Vanilla Ice Cream: Fat-Free, Regular	Vanilla Chocolate Swirl Ice Cream: Fat-Free, No Sugar Added, NutraSweet
Serving size	1/2 cup	1/2 cup
Total fat	0 grams	0 grams
Total carbohydrate	21 grams	21 grams
Equivalent in bread	1 1/2 slices of bread	1 1/2 slices of bread
Equivalent in pats of butter	0 pats of butter	0 pats of butter

In most cases, you'd think that this choice is a no-brainer. But, after you compare the nutrients on the label, you'll see that they will have about the same effect on your blood glucose levels.

6. **Watch out for fat-free foods.** When fat is reduced or totally removed from foods, the sugar and/or starch is usually increased to help keep the food's structure and texture the same and to enhance taste. Therefore, low-fat and fat-free foods are usually higher in carbohydrate. This does not mean that we need to avoid these foods; we just need to read the label carefully. Here's another example.

	Original Potato Chips	Baked Potato Chips
Serving size	1 ounce (12 chips)	1 ounce (12 chips)
Total fat	10 grams	2 grams
Total carbohydrate	15 grams	25 grams
Equivalent in bread	1 slice of bread	1 1/2 slices of bread
Equivalent in pats of butter	2 pats of butter	less than 1/2 pat of butter

As you can see here, if you choose the baked variety of potato chips, you are taking in less fat, but you will be taking in more carbohydrate. These are the choices you'll have to make when you purchase foods, so be prepared to carefully read the Nutrition Facts label.

COMMONLY ASKED QUESTIONS

I'm still confused about Net Carbs. Why is this term used on so many products today?

Low-carb diets have become very popular in recent years; however, most people are confused about how to lower their carbohydrate intake without totally losing the nutrients and healthy benefits from fruits, vegetables, grains, and legumes. We know that some carbohydrates are healthier choices than others. Processed and refined carbohydrates, such as white bread, white rice, mashed potatoes, and regular pasta, have been stripped of their healthy benefits: fiber and other nutrients. However, foods such as fresh fruits and vegetables, whole-grain breads, rice, pasta, cereals, and legumes are rich in fiber and nutrients and should be the foundation of any healthy diet. Although Net Carb is not an approved label term and neither is it necessary to buy only foods labeled as Low Carb, it is always important to look at the entire food label on any food before purchasing. Net Carbs are calculated by subtracting all of the dietary fiber from the total carbohydrate content of a food (and if the product contains more than 10 grams of sugar alcohols, one-half of the grams of sugar alcohols are deducted, too).

How can I lower my carbohydrate intake without purchasing only foods labeled Low Carb?

Actually, you can eat regular foods by focusing on plenty of nonstarchy vegetables and salads, choosing whole-grain rice and pasta, eating a baked potato with the skin, and selecting sweet potatoes instead of white potatoes. Buy whole-grain breads and cereals with at least 3 grams of fiber per serving, and limit sugar-free foods, which still contain carbohydrate and calories.

How much should my carbohydrate intake be reduced?

Carbohydrate needs are individualized for each person depending on age, activity, weight goals, and other health issues, such as heart or kidney disease. In 2002, the National Academy of Sciences recommended that adults get at least 130 grams of carbohydrate per day. This amount of carbohydrate is the *smallest* amount that is needed to adequately fuel your brain and nervous system. Before you decide to cut your carbohydrate intake, visit a registered dietitian who will guide you toward the proper amount for you as an individual.

YOUR TURN

Now it is your turn to recall some key points from this chapter. Let's see how you do!

1. All carbohydrate foods are created equal. True or false?

2. An adult should have no less than _____ grams of carbohydrate per day for proper brain and nervous system function.

3. When fat is reduced or totally removed from a product, it is often replaced by _____ or _____ to maintain the structure and texture of the food and to enhance taste.

4. Nutrition information on a Nutrition Facts label is always given on a per-serving basis. True or false?

See APPENDIX A for the answers.

CHAPTER 9

DIABETES AND BODY WEIGHT

> ## MYTH
>
> People with diabetes should lose a lot of weight in order to control their blood glucose levels.

ELAINE: I think I'd be able to control my diabetes and get off my medication if I could lose about 50 pounds.

DIETITIAN: It's true that losing weight, if you need to, can help you better manage your diabetes, blood pressure, and cholesterol levels. But some people still need to take medication for their diabetes, even if they're at a healthy weight.

ELAINE: Well, now that I have to take insulin, I find that it's a lot harder for me to lose weight than before I got diabetes. I've also heard that insulin causes you to gain weight, so it's probably going to be impossible for me to ever reach my ideal weight.

DIETITIAN: Losing weight can be hard for anyone, even for people who don't have diabetes. There is good news, though. First, just because you're on insulin doesn't mean you can't lose weight. Second, we know that losing even a small amount of weight, even as little as 10 pounds, can make a big difference in your diabetes management. You don't have to reach an "ideal" weight to reap the benefits of weight loss.

ELAINE: I didn't realize that. But shouldn't I try to get closer to my high school weight so I can get off insulin?

DIETITIAN: Actually, your goal should be to reach a weight that is realistic and healthy for you. Your goal isn't to necessarily get off insulin. Remember that any amount of weight loss is helpful, and you'll likely find that your blood glucose, along with your lipids and blood pressure, will improve. Plus, you'll feel better and breathe easier, too.

THE OLD AND THE NEW

Back in the days before insulin was discovered, the only treatment for diabetes was to put a person on a starvation diet. The theory was that the less a person with diabetes ate, the less his or her blood glucose would increase to unsafe levels. Although times have changed, the starvation approach to weight loss, unfortunately, still prevails. Many people, including health care professionals, believe that strict low-calorie diets are the only way to lose weight. It seems like every few years, a new kind of fad diet appears on the scene. Remember the grapefruit diet? How about the cabbage soup diet? How about those medically supervised diets consisting of 800 calories per day? Maybe you tried them and lost weight, but how long were you able to stay on the diet? Here's the million-dollar question: how long did you keep the weight off? The health care community has learned a lot over the past few decades about the best way to lose weight and keep that weight off. The days of starvation regimens should be a thing of the past because most of them don't work over the long term. Plus, many of these diets can be dangerous, particularly for people with certain conditions, such as diabetes.

You may be asking yourself, "Why should I even bother to lose weight, then? If diets don't work, how will

I ever lose weight?" Don't get discouraged. Fortunately, you don't have to resign yourself to being overweight. Studies have shown us that losing even a small amount of weight, such as 10 pounds, can make a real difference (for the better) in your diabetes. Some people with type 2 diabetes, like Elaine, may be able to either reduce their diabetes medication or come off of it altogether by losing weight and increasing physical activity. (This doesn't apply to people with type 1 diabetes, however. They will always have to take insulin, although they may be able to reduce their dose.)

Here Are the Facts

If you are overweight, or have been in the past, you know more than anyone how those extra pounds affect your whole body. You probably get tired very easily. You may quickly become short of breath. Your back, knees, or feet may hurt. You may even feel your heart pounding as you struggle to do the simplest chores. To make matters worse, if you have type 2 diabetes, being overweight makes it harder for your body to use its own insulin properly. It then becomes increasingly difficult to manage your blood glucose, and you end up taking more and more diabetes medication. Other health problems can stem from being overweight. Your blood pressure, cholesterol, and triglyceride levels can steadily creep up. No wonder your doctor keeps urging you to lose weight!

Diabetes and Insulin Resistance

Many people who have type 2 diabetes are advised to lose weight. Being overweight makes it difficult for insulin to do its job, which is to help lower and control blood glucose levels. Remember that insulin is a hormone that helps move glucose (sugar) from the bloodstream into cells to be used for energy. If someone is *resistant* to insulin, the glucose can't get into cells, no matter how much insulin is around. In fact, insulin levels in the blood often become high. This results from your pancreas producing more and more insulin in an effort to eventually make those cells "smarten up," so to speak, and let the glucose in.

Why does someone become insulin resistant? In two words: *abdominal fat*. If you have a roll of fat around your middle (also known as the "spare tire"), you have what is medically termed abdominal, or visceral, fat. This kind of fat is metabolically active in that it constantly releases fatty acids into the bloodstream, which, in turn, makes muscle cells less sensitive to insulin. These fatty acids can also infiltrate the liver, causing it to work less efficiently. To make matters worse, the liver starts to release more glucose and more lipoproteins (particles that carry cholesterol) into the blood. The combination of having too much abdominal fat, high blood glucose levels, high cholesterol, and high blood pressure has led some experts to label this as a syndrome, either the metabolic syndrome or cardiometabolic risk. No matter what you call it, if you have any or all of these risk factors, it can lead to serious health problems, especially heart disease. Fortunately, there are steps you can take to control these risk factors, including losing weight, controlling blood glucose levels, following a healthy eating plan, and being physically active on a regular basis. In some cases, medication may be needed, too.

Type 2 Diabetes

We know that most people with type 2 diabetes are overweight and thus are usually advised to lose some, if not all, of the excess weight. Remember, with type 2 diabetes, your body may still be producing insulin. The problem is that your insulin doesn't work very well. If you are able to lose a few pounds, your insulin actually starts to work better because your cells become more receptive (or less resistant) to your insulin. This means that your insulin can now do a better job of controlling your blood glucose levels. Another reason to lose weight if you have type 2 diabetes is that people with diabetes have twice the risk of developing heart disease. We know that being overweight increases your heart disease risk even further. Once again, the good news is that losing 10–20 pounds can help accomplish all this.

HERE'S WHAT YOU CAN DO

It's normal to feel overwhelmed and even discouraged when you try to lose weight, particularly if you've tried and failed in the past. While you secretly might hope to lose enough weight to look like a supermodel or a famous athlete, remember that you need to think realistically and practically. There's nothing wrong with wanting to look good, but it may help to focus first on the health benefits that come from losing a small amount of weight. Here are some ways to help you lose weight and help your diabetes (and your heart) at the same time.

1. Know Your Body Mass Index (BMI)

You might already be familiar with something called the body mass index or BMI for short. Throw away those old height and weight tables, which simply aren't realistic. How many five-foot, six-inch-tall men do you know who weigh 133 pounds? BMI is a more accurate way of figuring out your "fatness," so to speak, by evaluating your weight in relation to your height, because weight alone doesn't really gauge whether a person is overweight. (Picture one of your favorite NFL football players. He may be "overweight" according to height-weight tables, but most of his weight is probably muscle.) Look at the chart on p. 122 to find out how to calculate your BMI.

Calculate Your BMI

1. Multiply your weight in pounds by 703.
2. Divide the answer by your height in inches.
3. Divide again by your height in inches.

Let's follow an example. Let's say your height is 65 inches (5 feet, 5 inches) and your weight is 190 pounds.

1. $190 \times 703 = 133,570$
2. $133,570 \div 65 = 2,054.923$
3. $2,054.923 \div 65 = 31.6$, or 32

The BMI for this person is 32 kg/m².

What does that 32 mean? Here's how to interpret the numbers.

Weight Category	BMI
Underweight	Less than 18.5
Normal weight	18.5–24.9
Overweight	25–29.9
Obese	30 or higher

So, a BMI of 32, according to the definition, means that you are obese and that you should take some measures to lose weight. Fortunately, there are BMI charts readily available that have done the work for you (see p. 123–124). To use a BMI chart, find your height in feet and inches on the side and then your weight in pounds at the top. The number at which they intersect is your BMI.

Although health professionals often use BMI these days, remember that the one thing it can't tell you is your body fat percentage. This is something to consider when calculating and interpreting your BMI. Remember that

To use the table, find your height in the left-hand column labeled Height. Move across to your weight. The number at the top of the column is the BMI at that height and weight. Pounds have been rounded off.

BMI	19	20	21	22	23	24	25	26	27	28	29	30	31	32	33	34	35
Height (inches)							Body Weight (pounds)										
58	91	96	100	105	110	115	119	124	129	134	138	143	148	153	158	162	167
59	94	99	104	109	114	119	124	128	133	138	143	148	153	158	163	168	173
60	97	102	107	112	118	123	128	133	138	143	148	153	158	163	168	174	179
61	100	106	111	116	122	127	132	137	143	148	153	158	164	169	174	180	185
62	104	109	115	120	126	131	136	142	147	153	158	164	169	175	180	186	191
63	107	113	118	124	130	135	141	146	152	158	163	169	175	180	186	191	197
64	110	116	122	128	134	140	145	151	157	163	169	174	180	186	192	197	204
65	114	120	126	132	138	144	150	156	162	168	174	180	186	192	198	204	210
66	118	124	130	136	142	148	155	161	167	173	179	186	192	198	204	210	216
67	121	127	134	140	146	153	159	166	172	178	185	191	198	204	211	217	223
68	125	131	138	144	151	158	164	171	177	184	190	197	203	210	216	223	230
69	128	135	142	149	155	162	169	176	182	189	196	203	209	216	223	230	236
70	132	139	146	153	160	167	174	181	188	195	202	209	216	222	229	236	243
71	136	143	150	157	165	172	179	186	193	200	208	215	222	229	236	243	250
72	140	147	154	162	169	177	184	191	199	206	213	221	228	235	242	250	258
73	144	151	159	166	174	182	189	197	204	212	219	227	235	242	250	257	265
74	148	155	163	171	179	186	194	202	210	218	225	233	241	249	256	264	272
75	152	160	168	176	184	192	200	208	216	224	232	240	248	256	264	272	279
76	156	164	172	180	189	197	205	213	221	230	238	246	254	263	271	279	287

To use the table, find your height in the left-hand column labeled Height. Move across to your weight. The number at the top of the column is the BMI at that height and weight. Pounds have been rounded off.

Body Weight (pounds)

BMI / Height (inches)	36	37	38	39	40	41	42	43	44	45	46	47	48	49	50	51	52	53	54
58	172	177	181	186	191	196	201	205	210	215	220	224	229	234	239	244	248	253	258
59	178	183	188	193	198	203	208	212	217	222	227	232	237	242	247	252	257	262	267
60	184	189	194	199	204	209	215	220	225	230	235	240	245	250	255	261	266	271	276
61	190	195	201	206	211	217	222	227	232	238	243	248	254	259	264	269	275	280	285
62	196	202	207	213	218	224	229	235	240	246	251	256	262	267	273	278	284	289	295
63	203	208	214	220	225	231	237	242	248	254	259	265	271	276	282	287	293	299	304
64	209	215	221	227	232	238	244	250	256	262	267	273	279	285	291	296	302	308	314
65	216	222	228	234	240	246	252	258	264	270	276	282	288	294	300	306	312	318	324
66	223	229	235	241	247	253	260	266	272	278	284	291	297	303	309	315	322	328	334
67	230	236	242	249	255	261	268	274	280	287	293	299	306	312	319	325	331	338	344
68	236	243	249	256	262	269	276	282	289	295	302	308	315	322	328	335	341	348	354
69	243	250	257	263	270	277	284	291	297	304	311	318	324	331	338	345	351	358	365
70	250	257	264	271	278	285	292	299	306	313	320	327	334	341	348	355	362	369	376
71	257	265	272	279	286	293	301	308	315	322	329	337	343	351	358	365	372	379	386
72	265	272	279	287	294	302	309	316	324	331	338	346	353	361	368	375	383	390	397
73	272	280	288	295	302	310	318	325	333	340	348	355	363	371	378	386	393	401	408
74	280	287	295	303	311	319	326	334	342	350	358	365	373	381	389	396	404	412	420
75	287	295	303	311	319	327	335	343	351	359	367	375	383	391	399	407	415	423	431
76	295	304	312	320	328	336	344	353	361	369	377	385	394	402	410	418	426	435	443

Adapted from the National Heart, Lung, and Blood Institute (www.nhlbi.nih.gov/guidelines/obesity/bmi_tbl.htm).

solid, muscular football player? He may have a high BMI, maybe even putting him into the obese category, but most of his weight comes from muscle, not fat. On the other hand, someone may look slim and have a low BMI but may have more fat than muscle because he doesn't exercise. This person has an even higher risk of heart disease because he is more "fat" than "lean."

2. Know Your Waist Circumference

Another way to determine a healthy weight is by measuring your waist circumference. A large waist circumference means that you probably have too much abdominal fat. You can easily measure your waist circumference using a measuring tape. You have an increased risk of heart disease if your waist measures *more than 40 inches for men* or *more than 35 inches for women*. You should take steps to lose weight if you have a large waist circumference.

Once you know your BMI and your waist circumference, talk with your health care team about what to do next. Don't be discouraged if either your BMI or waist measurements are high. Instead, congratulate yourself for taking the first steps, and work with your team to develop a plan to get you the rest of the way.

3. Meet with a Registered Dietitian

All people with diabetes are encouraged to meet with a registered dietitian to develop a realistic meal plan. A good meal plan can help you not only control your blood glucose, but also help you lose and maintain weight. A meal plan should also provide you with a balance of foods and adequate nutrition. Maybe you've been handed a tear-off sheet for an 1,800-calorie diet by a well-meaning, but busy, doctor. This approach isn't very helpful for you because it's not personalized to the way you eat and the foods that you like. You need a plan that you can follow over the long term, and a dietitian is the team member who will help you develop this. He or she will determine how many calories you should be eating every day to lose weight gradually and safely. Your dietitian will also talk with you about what meal planning method will work best for you, whether it's using food choices (or exchanges), carbohydrate counting, or maybe even a combination of counting both carbohydrate and fat grams. The two of you, along with your physician, may decide that using a meal replacement for one or two meals each day is a good way to get you started with weight loss. Although we generally don't recommend fad diets, there are ways to customize certain kinds of these eating plans to work with your diabetes treatment plan under the supervision of your physician. So, you see that there are many options for meal planning. It's really a matter of finding out what will work best for you.

4. Learning to Eat Well

Below are some guidelines that will help you make healthy food choices to help you lose weight without going hungry. Remember, if you constantly feel hungry when trying to lose weight, you probably aren't eating enough calories. Therefore, your plan probably isn't realistic for you. Here are some things to keep in mind when putting together a realistic plan for eating well.

- **A calorie is a calorie is a calorie.** Despite what some health "experts" might have you believe, the bottom line for losing weight is to take in fewer calories than you normally do, while increasing your activity. Carbohydrate and protein contain 4 calories per gram, whereas fat contains 9 calories per gram. Obviously, it makes sense to first decrease your fat intake because calories from fat can quickly add up. But this doesn't mean you can expect to eat all the low-fat carbohydrate and protein foods you want, either. Too many calories from any source can lead to weight gain. By the way, alcohol contains 7 calories per gram, so it's a good idea to go easy with alcoholic beverages. Here's some food for thought: a pound of fat contains 3,500 calories.

Cutting back by 100 calories a day will lead to a 10-pound weight loss in one year! However, women should generally not consume fewer than 1,200 calories a day, and men should not have fewer than 1,500 calories a day unless it is done under medical supervision. If you're interested, you can figure out how many calories you're taking in, either by looking up your food choices in a calorie-counter book or by using tools available on the Internet. Another good option is to keep a record of your food intake for a week or so and then bring it to your dietitian, who can help you determine how many calories you are consuming and how to approach weight loss.

- **The pyramid or the plate?** Your dietitian should work with you to develop a plan for weight loss while making sure that you get all the nutrients that you need to stay healthy. As we've mentioned before, there are many tools available to help you—it's just a matter of finding out what suits you best. Together with your dietitian, you should develop your own eating plan that is customized to you and that you can follow. There are other options for meal planning, too. The USDA has a helpful, interactive tool called MyPyramid Plan. Check this out at www.MyPyramid.gov.

  If you're not quite ready for a structured eating plan, consider using an approach called the Plate Method. This is a simple, effective tool that can not only help you control your blood glucose levels, but can also help you with portion control. Here's how it works. Draw a circle the size of your plate on a piece of paper or take a paper or Styrofoam plate.

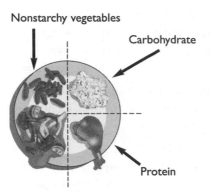

Nonstarchy vegetables

Carbohydrate

Protein

Next, draw a line right down the center of the plate. One-half of your plate should be filled with plenty of nonstarchy vegetables, such as broccoli, spinach, green beans, or carrots. Now, divide the second half of your plate in half again. Fill one-quarter with a carbohydrate food such as rice, pasta, or potato. The other quarter should be filled with a protein food (about four ounces), such as poultry, fish, or lean meat. Then, on the side of your plate, add a small piece of fruit, a glass of nonfat or low-fat milk, or a cup of low-fat yogurt.

By "staying within the lines" of your plate, you'll automatically control your portions and likely eat less. Of course, the catch here is to use a plate that's not much larger than nine inches in diameter. Whether you use the pyramid, the plate, or another method, aim to get most of your food choices from healthy plant foods, such as whole grains, legumes, fruits, and vegetables. Fewer of your food choices should come from protein, milk, and fat foods. However, don't eliminate any food group from your eating plan when you are trying to lose weight.

- **Focus on fat first.** We know all calories count, but it makes sense to cut back on fat first, which will automatically shave calories from your daily food intake. The first step to take is to reduce the amount of fat you add to foods. Adding foods such as butter or margarine, mayonnaise, oil, and salad dressings can increase the fat content of the healthiest foods. You may decide to choose lower-fat or even fat-free versions of these condiments (remember, they still contain calories and maybe some carbohydrate). The second step is to reduce your intake of foods that are naturally high in fat, such as red meats, luncheon meats, cheese, whole milk, potato chips, and ice cream (you'll be doing your heart a favor, too). Ask your dietitian for a list of high-fat foods if you're not sure what these are. Be sure to read Nutrition Facts labels for the Total Fat content of the things you're buying. A food with no more than 3 grams of fat per serving is considered a low-fat food. Third, change how you cook. Bake, broil, poach, or grill your foods instead of frying or cooking with a lot of oil or butter. Use cooking spray, broth, or water for sautéing or stir-frying.

- **Fill up on fiber.** High-fiber foods add bulk to your diet. This is a good thing because it means that you'll feel more full sooner. Foods high in fiber include whole-grain breads and cereals, fruits and vegetables, and legumes (dried beans and peas). Be sure to drink plenty of fluids when you increase your fiber intake to prevent constipation. (See Chapter 3.)

- **Water works wonders.** No, water doesn't magically wash away the pounds, but it may help you feel more full if you drink enough, which means that you might not eat as much. Remember, too, that water has no calories, carbohydrates, or fat, and it's a good substitute for snacking! Nutrition researchers don't agree on how much you should drink each day, but it certainly doesn't hurt to aim for at least eight 8-ounce glasses every day. Space that out over the course of a day, and it won't seem like much. Plus, you can drink seltzer water (unflavored or flavored with a non-caloric sweetener) or add lemon or lime to add some taste.

- **Get a perspective on portions.** Maybe you eat all the "right" foods, but if your portions are too large, losing weight will be hard for you. Eating too much of any food, even those low in calories or low in fat, will get in the way of your weight loss efforts. For these reasons, dust off that food scale and dig out your measuring cups and spoons. Weigh and measure your foods for a few days; you may be surprised at how much you're really eating. Practicing portion control at home will also help you when you eat away from home.

- **Eat more often.** What? Eat more than two or three times a day? How will you lose weight? Believe it or not, eating more frequently during the day can help in your efforts to not only lose weight, but also control your diabetes. By eating more frequently, your metabolism stays revved up and your blood glucose levels stay on a more even keel. The key, though, is to eat *smaller* amounts of *lower-fat, higher-fiber* foods. We're not talking about eating six huge, fatty meals. Talk with your dietitian if you think this approach might work for you (Chapter 12).

- **Eat breakfast.** Even if you can't or don't want to eat six small meals each day, there's now a lot of evidence that adults who skip breakfast make up for it at the end of the day (and into the night). Also, 95% of the people who are members of the National Weight Control Registry, a group of more than 5,000 people who have lost at least 30 pounds and kept the weight off for one year or more, eat breakfast every day. People who eat breakfast tend to take in fewer calories than those who do not eat breakfast. Data from the American Heart Association show that those who eat breakfast are between 35 and 50% less likely to become obese. But remember, the "breakfast of champions" doesn't consist of fried eggs, sausage, and bacon. Instead, aim for whole-grain cereal or toast, fresh fruit, nonfat or low-fat milk, and a heart-healthy fat, such as trans-fat-free margarine, peanut butter, or a small handful of nuts.

5. Change Your Behaviors

One of the hardest parts of any weight loss program is learning how to change the behaviors that led you to gain weight in the first place. We know that overeating and lack of exercise can add some pounds, but eating habits become ingrained over the years, and they can be hard to change. The good news is that any habit can be broken and new ones can be formed, although it takes time. Maybe you tend to eat when you watch TV; if so, try eating in a room without a TV, so you can break the connection between watching TV and eating. Perhaps you're an "emotional eater," which means that you eat when you're upset, depressed, or bored. If you are an emotional eater, then your goal is to take your mind off eating and get involved in other activities, such as going for a walk, cleaning the house, or calling a friend. Keep a record of when, why, and what you eat to help pinpoint problem areas that you need to focus on. If you find that you're struggling with this, consider joining a support group or seeking professional help.

6. Get Moving!

By now, you're probably aware that exercise and physical activity is very important for anyone with diabetes. If you have type 2 diabetes, regular activity will increase your sensitivity to insulin, which means that your blood glucose control will improve. Exercise lowers your risk for heart disease and some types of cancer. Exercise helps reduce stress, anxiety, and depression. Exercise is an absolute requirement if you are trying to lose weight or maintain weight loss. In fact, people who engage in regular physical activity are more likely to not regain the pounds they previously lost. Why is activity so important? Remember that exercise keeps your metabolism high. This means that you burn more calories, even when you're relaxing. Exercise does this by increasing your lean muscle mass and decreasing your fat mass. Muscle burns calories; fat doesn't. As people age, they tend to put on 10 pounds of fat per decade! But at the same time, they also lose muscle mass. The way to reverse this trend is to become and stay active. Once you reach your goal weight, being active for about one hour every day is critical for maintaining that weight loss. Although one hour of activity sounds like a lot, you don't have to do it all at once. It's okay to break it up over the course of the day. As you work with your dietitian on an eating plan, also consider meeting with an exercise physiologist, who can help design an activity program that is suited to you. (See Chapter 13 to learn more about exercise and physical activity).

Commonly Asked Questions

My doctor said I need to lose 50 pounds to help my diabetes. How will I ever lose this much?

Your doctor knows that losing weight will help you improve your diabetes management and reduce your risk of other diseases. However, losing this much weight can seem overwhelming. First, talk with your doctor or dietitian about a healthy weight that's realistic for you. Next, with your health care team, come up with a plan to lose your weight slowly and safely. Try breaking down your 50 pounds (or your target amount) into five-pound increments; in other words, work on losing just five pounds at a time. Aim for losing no more than one to two pounds of weight a week. Remember, losing even 10% of your weight will lead to health improvements.

I eat less now than I did when I was 25 years old, but I find that my weight keeps creeping up and up. What's going on?

Join the club. You're experiencing what happens to most people as they age: for every decade after the twenties, people tend to gain 10 pounds. Your metabolism has dropped, meaning that you're no longer burning calories like you used to. Although cutting back on your portion sizes will help, make sure you're getting a minimum of 30 minutes of activity at least five times a week and are including strength training as part of your routine. This will help boost your metabolism and eventually lead to weight loss.

Everything I eat is low fat. I don't add fat to food, and I don't cook with any fat. I also walk four times a week. Why can't I lose weight?

First, ask yourself how much you're eating of any food, low fat or otherwise. Maybe you really are consuming just a small amount of fat each day, but how much pasta, fruit, or chicken are you eating? Earlier, we discussed how large portions of any food can lead to weight gain, unless you're burning off those calories through exercise. First, try weighing and measuring your food portions and keeping a food record. This will help you see how much you're really eating. Next, sit down with a dietitian to work out a plan that will keep those portions under control. Finally, make sure you walk for at least 30 minutes (preferably every day) and add some strength training exercises to your routine to help build lean mass. An exercise physiologist can help you work out an activity plan.

I find I'm snacking a lot at night after dinner when I'm watching TV. I don't think I'm even hungry, but I can't seem to break this habit. This is wreaking havoc with my diabetes, and I've been gaining weight. What can I do?

Try not to keep high-fat, empty-calorie foods in your house. Even if you hide them away, you'll know they're there and will easily find them. If you must snack when watching TV, choose a low-calorie snack, such as raw vegetables or sugar-free Popsicles, or sip on water to help distract you from reaching for food. Take advantage of the commercials to get up and stretch or do a few exercises while you're watching your program. Finally, think about how much time you spend every day watching TV. Could you instead spend some of this time going for a walk, working out to an exercise DVD, or jogging on the treadmill? Break the habit of watching TV and eating by shaking up your routine.

YOUR TURN

Now it is your turn to recall some key points from this chapter. Let's see how you do!

1. Too much abdominal fat can increase your chances of getting heart disease. True or false?
2. You have to lose at least 30 pounds before your blood glucose levels will improve. True or false?
3. One simple meal planning approach that can help you lose weight and control your diabetes at the same time is called the _____ method.
4. List three steps you can take right now to help you lose weight:

   _____

   _____

   _____

5. Figure out your body mass index (BMI) and waist circumference.

   BMI: _____ kg/m^2

   Waist circumference: _____ inches

   Recalculate your measurements in one to three months and see how you're doing!

See APPENDIX A for the answers.

CHAPTER 10

DIABETES AND THE USE OF SUPPLEMENTS

> ## MYTH
>
> People with diabetes should take special dietary supplements.

JULIE: Should I be taking this diabetic vitamin supplement? I get so confused. I don't know what to take. I read and hear about all these special vitamins and supplements that are supposed to be good for people with diabetes.

DIETITIAN: It certainly can be confusing for *anyone* these days, because there's more and more research coming out about what we need to stay healthy and possibly prevent disease. Many manufacturers of dietary supplements market "special" supplements to people with diabetes.

JULIE: But don't they help? Or is it all just a waste of money?

DIETITIAN: Some may be helpful, but others might even be harmful. There's not a lot of good evidence that supplements will improve your diabetes management or help you prevent complications. The most important thing is that you eat a healthful diet, especially one that contains a lot of vegetables, fruits, and whole-grain foods. If your eating plan isn't well balanced, popping supplements isn't going to help much.

Foods contain many other substances that you just can't get in pill form.

JULIE: But sometimes I just don't have time to eat healthily every day. Should I be taking *any* supplements?

DIETITIAN: That's a good question. Let's take a closer look at what you're eating and what you might need in the way of a supplement.

What's Next?

Can you identify with Julie? It seems like every day, researchers learn more and more about nutrition, especially about vitamins, minerals, and other types of supplements. If you pick up a newspaper or magazine or simply turn on the TV, there's sure to be a story about the latest vitamin you should be taking or food you should be eating more often. If you walk down the aisles of a drug store, health food store, or local supermarket, the rows and rows of bottles can become overwhelming. But what do we really need to take to stay healthy and prevent disease? Do people with diabetes really need special supplements?

The Old and the New

Chances are, your parents or grandparents didn't take vitamin supplements when they were young. Many supplements either hadn't been discovered or not much was known about them. The supplements that did exist were mostly used to treat vitamin deficiencies, such as scurvy.

These days, the supplement industry is big business. Americans spend $7 billion per year on various supplements. According to a survey by the National Nutritional Foods Association in 2002, more than 242 million Americans take supplements, such as vitamins, minerals, herbal remedies, or other specialty products. Fifty-two percent of

Americans take multivitamin supplements. Seven out of 10 Americans take supplements because they make them feel better, and 67% take them to prevent illness. Almost 60% of Americans take supplements to help them build muscle mass.

On the other hand, many people are hesitant to take supplements. Here are some of the reasons they give for not taking supplements.

- They are unsure what to take.
- They feel that supplements cost too much.
- Their doctors don't recommend them.
- They think supplements are unsafe.
- They can get the nutrients they need from the food they eat.

The last point is interesting. For many years the medical profession often scoffed at the idea that people needed to take supplements, unless there was a clear need for them, such as taking an iron supplement for anemia. They claimed that people should get all of the nutrients they need from food (which still isn't a bad idea). Another reason for their skepticism was that not a lot was known about what people should take, how much they should take, and what possible harmful side effects certain supplements could induce. Today, we know more, even enough to start to make some concrete recommendations on supplement use.

In this chapter, we'll examine some of the more popular supplements touted for diabetes and the pros and cons of each. Before we go any further, however, please note that the information presented in this chapter is not meant to serve as medical advice. You should always discuss supplement use with your doctor or dietitian because taking the wrong type or too much of any supplement may be harmful.

WHAT ARE SUPPLEMENTS AND WHAT DO THEY DO?

Let's first make sure you know what we mean when we casually chat about vitamins, minerals, and dietary supplements.

Vitamins come from living materials, such as plants and animals. They are needed in very small amounts to

- process the food we eat
- help form blood cells
- help form DNA (genetic material)
- help form hormones
- assist enzymes in their various jobs

There are a total of 13 vitamins. They can be categorized as either *water soluble* or *fat soluble*. Water-soluble vitamins are not stored in the body. They include the B vitamins and vitamin C. Fat-soluble vitamins require fat to be absorbed and are stored in the fat tissue. These include vitamins A, D, E, and K. Although vitamins do not provide calories—like carbohydrate, protein, and fat—they do help the body convert calories into fuel for energy. Vitamins often work in conjunction with minerals to maintain good health.

A **mineral** is an inorganic substance that is involved in numerous functions in the body. These functions that use minerals include

- muscle contraction
- blood formation
- bone formation
- electrolyte balance
- nerve-impulse conduction
- energy production

Minerals are classified as being either *major*, meaning that they are found in the body in larger amounts, or *trace*, meaning that they are needed in very small amounts. The major minerals include calcium, magnesium, potassium, phosphorus, chloride, sodium, and sulfur. Trace minerals include iron, zinc, chromium, copper, and iodine. The major and trace minerals exist in the body in a careful balance with one another. So, if you take in a lot of one mineral, then that may interfere with the absorption of another and possibly result in a deficiency.

Dietary supplements include vitamins, minerals, antioxidants, amino acids, fatty acids, enzymes, fibers, herbs, steroids, and plant and animal substances (for example, shark cartilage). If you've ever looked for any specific supplement in your drug store, health food store, or supermarket, you've probably already seen that there is a supplement out there for anything and everything. Before we start buying, though, we need to ask ourselves whether we need these supplements and, if so, which ones? Should we pop a vitamin to make up for a lack of nutrients in our diets? What about disease prevention? There are several things you need to consider before you swallow that fistful of pills, including safety, effectiveness, and cost. The best way to find out what is right for you is to discuss this issue with your health care team first.

Antioxidants

Antioxidants are substances that neutralize, or inactivate, free radicals. Free radicals are troublemakers. They are unstable oxygen molecules that damage cells, which in turn can lead to diseases (such as cancer, heart disease, nerve diseases, and cataracts) and premature aging. Free radicals are formed from environmental factors such as tobacco smoke, pollution, ultraviolet light, and X-rays and by the body's metabolism. By neutralizing free radicals, antioxidants can prevent much of the damage caused by these harmful molecules. There are actually many antioxidants; some are vitamins, some are minerals, and some are even plant substances. We'll review the main ones that have been linked to diabetes.

Vitamin C

Vitamin C is a water-soluble vitamin with known antioxidant effects. Some studies show that vitamin C can help fight heart attacks, strokes, cancer, and cataracts. There is some debate as to whether people really need to take vitamin C from dietary supplements because there are so many foods rich in this vitamin. Eating several servings of fruits and vegetables each day can ensure that you're getting at least the RDA (Recommended Dietary Allowance) for this vitamin, which is 90 milligrams for men and 75 milligrams for women. Many people swear by this vitamin to either prevent or lessen the severity of colds, although no good scientific research has been able to support this common thought.

How might vitamin C affect diabetes? People with diabetes tend to have lower levels of vitamin C in their bodies, which may be due to high blood glucose levels reducing the amount of vitamin C that is taken into cells. However, vitamin C may be linked to diabetes in yet another way. It's well documented that people with diabetes have a higher risk of developing cardiovascular disease than people without diabetes, and some research has shown that taking vitamin C regularly can reduce the chances of developing heart disease. However, even though people with diabetes often have low levels of vitamin C, taking high doses may actually cause the same cardiovascular damage as high glucose levels. While researchers continue to debate about the pros and cons of taking vitamin C supplements, most would agree that getting vitamin C from foods is safe. There is a risk that taking this vitamin in supplement form may upset the balance of the body's antioxidants and pro-oxidants.

Until we learn more about the role of vitamin C and its effects in people with diabetes, it's wise to aim to meet your daily requirement through food sources.

Vitamin E

If ever a vitamin were to give the science of nutrition a bad name, that vitamin would be vitamin E. It wasn't too long ago that researchers couldn't say enough good things about this antioxidant, touting its role in the prevention of heart disease. The celebrations abruptly stopped in 2000 after data were released from a study called, ironically, the HOPE (Heart Outcomes Prevention Evaluation) study. After tracking almost 10,000 men and women aged 55 or older who took either vitamin E or a placebo for five years, those who took vitamin E had just as many strokes, heart attacks, and deaths from heart disease as those who took the placebo. Shortly after this study was released, another study reported that 11,000 patients who had had a heart attack and took 300 international units (IU) of vitamin E were slightly more likely to have a second heart attack than those taking a placebo. In 2004, after reviewing findings from 14 studies, the American Heart Association reported that taking 400 IU or more of vitamin E increased the risk of death.

However, other evidence shows just the opposite for people with diabetes. Using the data from the same HOPE study, researchers found that people with diabetes who took vitamin E reduced their risk of heart attack by 43% and their risk of dying from heart disease by 55%. At least one study shows that vitamin E may help prevent the onset of type 2 diabetes.

The recommended daily intake for vitamin E is 15 milligrams (22.5 IU) for both men and women over the age of 14, which is easily obtainable through food sources or by taking a multivitamin. Although some studies show that 400 IU may be the amount required for optimal health, scientists caution against taking high doses of this vitamin, as it may lead to an increased risk of bleeding, especially in people who take aspirin or other blood thinners. Until we learn more about vitamin E, it's best to aim for getting your vitamin E from food sources and a multivitamin.

Here's the Scoop: Vitamin E

Role: helps form red blood cells, muscle, and tissue; involved in cell metabolism

Food sources: sunflower seeds, nuts, wheat germ, vegetable oils

Recommended daily amount: 15 mg (22.5 IU)

Possible harm: large amounts may increase the risk of stroke in people with high blood pressure; may interfere with medication that prevents blood clots

---

B Vitamins

The B vitamins are actually a cluster of several different vitamins (there is no "vitamin B," by the way). The B vitamins include folic acid, B12, thiamin, riboflavin, niacin, B6, and pantothenic acid. All of these vitamins are involved in helping the body obtain energy from food. Folic acid plays an important role in preventing birth defects. Vitamin B12 helps keep nerves healthy. Niacin, used in large doses as a prescription medication, can help lower cholesterol levels.

In more recent years, a link has been established between an amino acid called homocysteine and a risk for heart disease and stroke. It's thought that high levels of homocysteine can damage the lining of arteries and trigger blood clots. Some studies show that people with type 2 diabetes with high homocysteine levels have a higher risk of death from heart disease.

Three of the B vitamins—folic acid, vitamin B6, and vitamin B12—can help break down homocysteine in the body into nontoxic substances. However, no good studies have shown that taking B vitamin supplements actually lowers the risk of heart disease or death from heart disease, even though the supplements can lower homocysteine levels. Until we learn more about the connections among homocysteine, B vitamins, and heart disease, the American Heart Association doesn't recommend that people take B vitamin supplements, but does encourage people to obtain their B vitamins from food sources, including leafy green vegetables, fruit, legumes, and wheat germ, for example.

Here's the Scoop: B Vitamins

Recommended daily amount:

Folic acid:	400 micrograms
Vitamin B6:	1.3–1.7 mg
Vitamin B12:	2.4 micrograms

Possible harm: nerve damage; itching, gastrointestinal symptoms; high doses can mask the symptoms of certain types of anemia

---

Minerals

Magnesium

There is a definite link between diabetes and magnesium. Magnesium helps the pancreas secrete insulin. If a person does not have enough magnesium, then he or she does not have enough insulin around to control blood glucose levels. Studies have shown that people who don't get enough magnesium in their diets have a higher risk of developing type 2 diabetes. In addition, a high percentage of people who already have type 2 diabetes have low magnesium levels, although it's hard to say which came first, the diabetes or the low magnesium levels. People with diabetes can lose magnesium in their urine if their blood glucose levels are poorly controlled. Diuretics (drugs for controlling blood pressure or fluid retention) can also result in a loss of magnesium from the body. Other people at risk for low magnesium include those who have congestive heart failure, heart attacks, diabetic ketoacidosis, calcium or potassium deficiencies, and pregnant women. Magnesium may help prevent some of the complications associated with diabetes, such as eye disease and heart disease. However, no evidence shows that taking magnesium supplements improves blood glucose levels because so many other factors are involved in blood glucose management.

Here's the Scoop: Magnesium

Role: involved with energy production; aids in muscle contraction, heartbeat regulation, and nerve transmission; needed for insulin secretion; may help prevent heart disease, stroke, osteoporosis and migraines

Food sources: whole-grain breads and cereals, legumes, nuts, bananas, leafy green vegetables

Recommended daily amount: 320 mg for women; 420 mg for men

Possible harm: diarrhea, drowsiness, lethargy, impaired calcium absorption

---

Chromium

Chromium, in the form of chromium picolinate, has been in the spotlight for a while because of claims that this trace mineral can reduce body fat and build muscle, yet no good evidence exists that chromium is effective as a weight-loss aid or as a muscle builder. However, chromium may play a role in the management of diabetes. Chromium is a trace mineral needed for metabolism and to produce glucose tolerance factor, which helps insulin to work efficiently. Several studies over the past 30 years show that chromium may help improve blood glucose levels as well as lipid (cholesterol and triglyceride) levels. In addition, evidence suggests that chromium may play a role in other conditions, such as reducing the risk of heart attack, glaucoma, and bone loss.

Unfortunately, it's very difficult to both reliably measure blood chromium levels and to predict the response to chromium supplementation in people with diabetes. Researchers also do not know how much chromium we really need and how much is in the foods we eat, which makes it difficult to even recommend a supplement dosage. Fortunately, this mineral is relatively safe, and recent research concerning chromium supplementation and diabetes control looks promising.

If you decide to try chromium as a supplement, first discuss this with your health care team. Chromium can negatively interact with some medications, including insulin, beta-blockers, and antacids. Don't take any more

---

Here's the Scoop: Chromium

Role: aids in the metabolism of carbohydrate and fat; component of glucose tolerance factor

Food sources: brewer's yeast, whole-grain breads and cereals, orange juice, wine

Adequate intake amount: 20–35 micrograms, up to 1,000 micrograms with a doctor's consent

Possible harm: possible kidney and chromosome damage in extremely high amounts

than 400–800 micrograms of chromium per day and be sure to check your blood glucose levels regularly.

Cinnamon

You need look no further than your kitchen cabinet for a spice that may truly help you lower your blood glucose and lipid levels. Cinnamon, a popular spice used to season many different foods, is a dietary supplement that has been gaining in popularity over the past few years. This spice contains antioxidants called phenols, which are substances that may help control glucose levels and lower the risk of heart disease. There's also another natural substance in cinnamon, called polyphenol, which may have insulin-like properties. A study involving people with type 2 diabetes who were given various doses of cinnamon (one, three, or six grams) showed beneficial effects. All doses of cinnamon lowered fasting glucose, LDL cholesterol, total cholesterol, and triglyceride levels.

Cinnamon is considered to be quite safe, with no significant harmful side effects, other than possibly causing an allergic reaction in certain individuals. However, researchers aren't ready to make a recommendation regarding if and how much cinnamon a person should take. As always, proceed with caution before taking any kind of supplement. Talk to your health care provider if you'd like to try cinnamon, start with the lowest effective dose (1 gram or 1/5 teaspoon), and be sure to monitor your blood glucose levels carefully.

HERE'S WHAT YOU CAN DO

Now you might be asking yourself, "Do I need a supplement? If so, which one or ones? And how much?"

First of all, there are certain groups of people who may need one or more supplements for vitamins or minerals. Who are they and what might they need?

- **Women:** may need calcium, iron, folic acid
- **Adolescents:** may need calcium, iron, multivitamin/mineral
- **Seniors:** may need multivitamin/mineral, calcium, vitamin D, vitamin B12
- **Vegetarians:** may need calcium, vitamin D, iron, vitamin B12
- **Smokers:** may need vitamin C

In fact, almost anyone could potentially benefit from taking a supplement if his or her diet is less than optimal. With all of the studies and reports coming out about how a particular vitamin may prevent a particular disease or condition, many people have started taking supplements for this very reason. Below are some guidelines to help you make an informed decision.

1. **The first step.** Sit down with a dietitian. Do you skip meals? Dislike fruits and vegetables? Never drink milk? A dietitian is uniquely qualified to thoroughly assess your current eating plan, tell you what you're missing, and help you improve. Generally, the first and wisest step is to obtain any missing nutrients from food sources; if that's not possible, or if you're not willing to, she or he may suggest that you take either a multivitamin or an individual supplement.

2. **Where to begin?** Start with a multivitamin/mineral supplement. Even choosing this can be daunting! Your best bet is to pick a multivitamin with no more than 100–150% of the Daily Value for the listed vitamins and minerals (there should be at least 20 on the label). Make sure it contains 400 micrograms of folic acid and 400 IU of vitamin D. If you're a man, you may want to pick a supplement without iron.

3. **Additives, colors, and fillers...oh my!** Unless you have a particular intolerance or allergy to a coloring or filler ingredient, such as lactose, don't

worry about these ingredients in supplements. They may actually help with absorption. You'll simply pay more for a supplement without them.

4. **Choose well-known brands.** Recent research conducted by ConsumerLab.com, an independent evaluator of health and nutrition products, revealed that several brands of multivitamins failed to meet quality standards, and some were even contaminated with lead. Other supplements failed to dissolve within the 30-minute standard set by the U.S. Pharmacopeia. The keys to choosing safe and effective multivitamins and mineral supplements are to purchase well-known brands, to purchase supplements from reputable retailers (rather than from unknown sellers on the Internet, for example), and to look on the bottle for a seal from the US Pharmacopeia, ConsumerLab.com, or NSF.

5. **Natural versus synthetic.** These days, anything that says "natural" has got to be better, right? Not always, at least when it comes to vitamins and minerals. Natural and synthetic supplements are identical and will work in your body the same way. It's also less expensive to produce synthetic vitamins; therefore, you end up saving money by purchasing synthetic ones. However, natural vitamin E (D-alpha tocopherol) is actually better absorbed than its synthetic cousin, DL-alpha tocopherol.

6. **Healthy bones.** Unless you're either drinking at least three 8-ounce glasses of milk or eating about three 8-ounce containers of yogurt a day, you're probably short of calcium and should consider taking a supplement. Try to take your calcium in the form of calcium carbonate, which is highly concentrated. If you become gassy or constipated, take a form called calcium citrate. Either way, take at least 1,000 milligrams worth of tablets every day (the amount of calcium in supplements will vary).

Also, for better absorption, split your dosage over two or three meals, ideally taking no more than 500 milligrams at a time. If you rarely see the sun or are not drinking enough milk, take a calcium supplement with added vitamin D. Be sure to choose a supplement with the letters "USP" on the label. This means that the supplement meets the U.S. Pharmacopeia's standards for dissolution.

7. **Antioxidants.** Taking antioxidants, such as vitamins C, E, and beta carotene, is more controversial than taking a multivitamin. There's no conclusive evidence that antioxidants are beneficial for people with diabetes. However, if you decide to take them, take no more than 1,000 milligrams of vitamin C and no more than 400 IU of vitamin E daily.

8. **With or without food?** Supplements are best taken with food because they are better absorbed and will be available when carbohydrate, protein, and fat are digested. The fat-soluble vitamins (A, D, E, and K) need some fat for absorption, so these should definitely be taken with food.

9. **Expired?** Supplements will lose their potency over time, so throw out any supplements that have passed their expiration date. Also, keep your supplements away from heat, light, and moisture.

10. **Too much of a good thing?** Don't go overboard! Never take mega-doses of any supplement without first consulting with your health care team. Use the guidelines in this chapter to help you. At high doses, vitamins, minerals, and other supplements can act like medications and may be harmful.

11. **Other considerations.** If you are pregnant, elderly, or have certain health or medical conditions (including diabetes), talk with your health care provider *before* you take any supplement. Remember, *always* tell your provider what you are taking at *every* appointment.

SUMMARY

We hope this chapter has helped you sort out the often confusing world of supplements. As we learn more and more about supplements and nutrition in general, the guidelines above may change; this is inevitable when it comes to nutrition. This is why your health care team should be your partner in working with you to improve your eating and decide with you which, if any, dietary supplements you may need. Once again, remember that the ideal situation is to get your nutrients from food sources whenever possible. Eating according to the Dietary Guidelines and MyPyramid can help you make healthful food choices. Use vitamins, minerals, and supplements for what they really are...supplements, not substitutes.

YOUR TURN

Now it is your turn to recall some key points from this chapter. Let's see how you do!

1. Vitamins and minerals contain calories and give us energy. True or false?

2. Name an example of an antioxidant:

   _____

3. Cinnamon may help lower blood glucose levels in people with type 2 diabetes. True or false?

4. List two food sources for magnesium:

   _____.

   _____.

See APPENDIX A for the answers.

CHAPTER 11

SODIUM

> ## MYTH
>
> People with diabetes should be on a low-sodium diet.

DIETITIAN: How are things going with the meal plan we worked out last month?

KEVIN: Good, except that I think I'm eating too much sodium, and I know it's important to avoid using salt and eating salty foods.

DIETITIAN: You seem to be quite concerned about your sodium intake. Any particular reason why?

KEVIN: Well, I was told that people with diabetes shouldn't have sodium in their diets. This has been hard for me, because foods don't taste the same without salt.

DIETITIAN: Unless your doctor wants you to cut back on sodium because of your blood pressure or other medical conditions, some sodium is okay, although you don't want to go overboard. You're wise to be aware of sodium, though. If you do need to cut back on salt, there are ways to make food taste better by using herbs and spices instead of salt.

WHAT'S NEXT?

Like Kevin, many people who have diabetes believe that they need to restrict their sodium intake, whether they have hypertension (high blood pressure) or not. The truth is that although some people probably should be careful of the amount of high-sodium foods they ingest, salt and sodium have nothing to do with blood glucose control. If you have diabetes and your health care provider has recommended that you watch your sodium intake, it's most likely because you either have high blood pressure or are prone to retaining fluid in your body, but not because your blood glucose levels are running too high or too low.

THE OLD AND THE NEW

Mention the words "salt" or "sodium" to almost anyone these days and he or she will likely tell you that everyone needs to follow a low-sodium diet or that he or she is confused about the whole topic. For years, health authorities, including the U.S. Department of Agriculture and the American Heart Association, have been telling us that we need to cut back on salt because salt can raise blood pressure, which in turn increases our chances of having a heart attack or a stroke. Researchers have been debating for decades about the role of salt in blood pressure control. For example, should everyone limit his or her sodium intake or just people with high blood pressure? Does eating a high-sodium diet raise blood pressure and eating a low-sodium diet lower blood pressure? These are questions of extreme interest that are hot topics among the scientific community as well as at office coffee breaks.

Although the Salt Institute—a nonprofit trade association of salt producers—cites several studies on its website that report no significant health benefits from following a lower-sodium diet, most health authorities agree that it's a good idea to be on the safe side; even people with normal blood pressure levels should go easy on how much sodium they consume.

What Is Sodium and Why Do We Need It?

We tend to use the terms "salt" and "sodium" interchangeably, but they are not really the same. Salt is actually a chemical made up of about 40% sodium and 60% chloride, and sodium is an essential mineral that we need to survive. Sodium regulates blood pressure and blood volume and is also important in the contraction of muscles and the conduction of nerve impulses. Chloride is another mineral that helps conduct the flow of water in and out of cells. The kidneys carefully and tightly control sodium levels in the body. Too much sodium in the body can cause fluid retention, and too little sodium may lead to dehydration. Fortunately, our kidneys can get rid of any extra sodium that we take in through our diets, as long as they are working properly.

Although most of us need to be careful not to take in too much sodium, there are people, such as athletes or people who perspire heavily, who need to make sure they take in enough sodium. Symptoms of sodium deficiency are muscle cramps, dizziness, exhaustion, and even convulsions and death. Luckily, it's pretty easy to replenish sodium stores—just eat some salty foods and drink enough fluids that don't contain caffeine.

Where Is Sodium Found?

Sodium is found in all foods. However, we do not get most of our sodium by adding salt to foods at the dinner table or from foods in which sodium occurs naturally. Most of the sodium in our foods is added during processing. In fact, about 77% of the sodium that we ingest each day comes from processed foods and restaurant foods, which, not surprisingly, contain quite a bit of this mineral. You might wonder why food manufacturers add so much sodium to foods. One obvious reason is flavor. Sodium also makes food last longer by drawing moisture out of food, which limits the growth of any bacteria. Other reasons for increasing the sodium content of processed foods is that sodium can add thickness or bulk; it can mask any chemical aftertaste; and believe it or not, sodium can enhance the sweetness of foods, such as cakes and cookies.

Although some foods have an obvious salty taste—such as pretzels, pickles, and soy sauce—you may be surprised to learn that some of your favorite foods may contain quite a lot of sodium. Here are some examples.

- Canned soup
- Barbecue sauce
- Catsup
- Mustard
- Cereal
- Luncheon meats
- Cheese
- Salad dressing

Hidden sources of sodium can be uncovered by reading the ingredient list on a food package.

Some Examples of High-Sodium Ingredients

monosodium glutamate or MSG (flavor enhancer)

sodium benzoate (preservative)

sodium caseinate (thickener and binder)

sodium citrate (controls acidity in soft drinks)

sodium nitrite (curing agent in processed meats)

sodium phosphate (emulsifier, stabilizer)

sodium proprionate (mold inhibitor)

sodium saccharin (artificial sweetener)

baking soda

baking powder

THE UPSIDE AND THE DOWNSIDE OF SODIUM

You've already learned about the importance of sodium in the body. Remember that this mineral helps regulate blood pressure, muscle contraction, and transmission of nerve impulses. When your body is properly functioning, sodium keeps your fluid balance in control.

By now, you're most likely aware that sodium and high blood pressure don't mix. But what if you have normal blood pressure? Or what if your blood pressure is "borderline"? Should you cut back on your sodium intake in these cases?

The Scoop on Salt

Most Americans like the taste of salty foods. Try eating unsalted potato chips or pretzels. Not so tasty, are they? Corn on the cob just isn't the same without a liberal shaking of salt, either. Yet while we may indulge ourselves in our passion for salty foods, we usually do so with a feeling of guilt. Salt is bad for us, right? Sodium has been associated with high blood pressure for a long time. Doctors and other health care professionals usually advise their patients with high blood pressure to follow a low-sodium diet, often in conjunction with prescribing medications to control blood pressure. What is the connection? Let's learn a little about blood pressure, first.

A Blood Pressure Primer

Blood pressure refers to the force of blood pushing against artery walls as it flows through the body. Blood pressure can change many times over the course of the day and will go up, particularly if you're scared, upset, or if you're exercising. Blood pressure tends to drop when you are relaxing or sleeping. When your blood pressure is measured, the reading will appear as two numbers. The first number, which is the higher of the two, is the *systolic* pressure. This is the peak force of blood as it is forced through your arteries by the pumping of your heart. The second number, the *diastolic* pressure, is the force of blood when your heart is relaxing between beats and filling up with blood for the next beat.

Optimal blood pressure is a reading of less than 120 over 80, usually written like a fraction: 120/80. The goal for most people with diabetes is a blood pressure less than 130/80. A blood pressure reading of 140/90 is considered hypertension (or high blood pressure). There's also a newer category of hypertension now, called *prehypertension*, that is designated by a blood pressure of 120 to 139 over 80 to 89 (that is, between 120/80 and 139/89). People with prehypertension are at risk of developing high blood pressure, but the good news is that these folks can prevent getting high blood pressure by making healthy lifestyle changes, such as controlling their weight, eating a healthful diet, and getting regular physical activity.

Approximately 60 million people in the U.S. have high blood pressure, and it is about 50% more common in African Americans than in Caucasians. This may be due in part to the fact that African Americans have a higher amount of aldosterone in the body. Aldosterone is a hormone that promotes sodium retention. In addition, high blood pressure is more common in Hispanics and in people with diabetes, kidney problems, and a family history of high blood pressure. Other risk factors for high blood pressure include excess weight, tobacco use, lack of exercise, stress, and alcohol consumption.

High blood pressure is the most common of all the cardiovascular (heart) diseases. Untreated high blood pressure forces the heart to work consistently harder, leading to damage of the blood vessels, brain, eyes, and kidneys. It is the leading cause of stroke and one of the three main risk factors for having a heart attack (the other two are smoking and high blood cholesterol). So far, there is no cure for high blood pressure, but it can be controlled with medication and/or lifestyle changes.

The scary thing about high blood pressure is that there are few, if any, symptoms. Many people with high blood pressure do not even know they have it, giving this disease the label of "silent killer." Another scary fact is that of those people who have high blood pressure, 71% don't have it under control. The effects of untreated high blood pressure can be deadly. Half a million people die each year from complications relating to high blood pressure. High blood pressure takes a monetary toll, as well. According to the American Heart Association, the economic cost of high blood pressure (a measure of the total cost on a society of a disease or condition, including health care costs, hours of work lost, and so forth) in 2006 was an astounding $63.5 billion.

What's the Connection?

So how does sodium fit into all of this? Believe it or not, people have been advised to watch their sodium intake since 2500 B.C., when Chinese physicians warned their patients to use less salt or else their pulses would harden. Since then, scientists have determined that the higher the salt intake of a population, the greater the incidence of high blood pressure. No one is exactly sure how sodium affects blood pressure, but it may be that too much salt in the diet damages sodium channels (which move sodium in and out of cells). Over time, the kidneys have a tougher time trying to flush excess sodium out of the body and blood pressure starts to climb.

Most of the information linking a high sodium intake to high blood pressure originates from 1988 data from the Intersalt Study. This study looked at approximately 10,000 men and women of all ages from different countries. The researchers found that the higher the sodium intake, the higher the blood pressure and that blood pressure rises with increasing age in cultures that eat a high-sodium diet. They then concluded that a high-sodium diet causes high blood pressure.

Other studies since the Intersalt Study have led to similar conclusions. The Trials of Hypertension Prevention (TOHP II) showed that adults with prehypertension who decreased their sodium intake by about 900 milligrams per day lowered their blood pressure by 1.7 over 0.9 points (that is, 1.7/0.9). The Trial of Nonpharmacologic Interventions in the Elderly (TONE) also looked at older adults with prehypertension who cut their daily sodium intake by 25%. Their blood pressure dropped by 2.6 over 1.1 points (2.6/1.1). Another key study that has gotten much recognition by the media is the Dietary Approaches to Stop Hypertension (DASH) study. In this study, more than 400 people followed a diet with either 3,300 (high), 2,400 (medium), or 1,500 milligrams (low) of sodium for one month. Those who went from the high- to low-sodium diet lowered their blood pressure by 6.7 over 3.5 points (6.7/3.5). The group that ate what is now known as the DASH diet (high in fruits, vegetables, and low-fat dairy foods) lowered their blood pressure by an average of 3.0 over 1.6 points (3.0/1.6). Although the drop in blood pressure in these studies may seem trivial, the health impact of lowering blood pressure by even just a few points is enormous.

The bottom line is that cutting back on your sodium intake is helpful in decreasing and controlling blood pressure. Yet despite all of the evidence pointing to the benefits of lowering sodium intake, many people in the U.S. continue to eat at least 4,000 milligrams of sodium on a daily basis. There are many reasons why people don't lower their sodium intake, including the fact that most people believe that simply not adding salt to their food is sufficient, even though we know that most of our sodium intake comes from processed foods and restaurant foods.

Adding to this complicated situation is the fact that many people who have normal blood pressure readings don't believe that they should lower their sodium intake. Unfortunately, some of these same people may have what is known as "salt sensitivity." In someone who is salt sensitive, his or her blood pressure greatly increases after eating a high-sodium meal. Studies show that being salt sensitive can increase the risk of death as much as having high blood pressure. There's no easy way to diagnose someone who is salt sensitive, but there are steps you can take to find out if you have it. First, get your blood pressure checked at least twice a year and keep a record of your readings. Look for any upward trends in your blood pressure. You might even want to monitor your blood pressure at home to learn how eating more or less sodium affects your readings. Second, review your family's medical history for high blood pressure or heart disease. Third, pay attention to how your clothes, shoes, and socks fit after eating a high-sodium meal. If your socks are cutting into your legs or your shoes feel tight, you may be retaining fluid, a possible sign of salt sensitivity. Also keep in mind that you may have normal blood pressure now but that it's always possible that it will climb up as you get older. The key, therefore, is to focus on *preventing* high blood pressure in the first place.

Other Problems with a High Sodium Intake

High blood pressure is the primary medical problem linked to a diet high in salt. However, there are other physical effects linked to a high sodium intake. For example, there is some evidence that a high-sodium diet can be a risk factor for osteoporosis, stomach cancer, and even asthma. So, although you may have normal blood pressure, it may be prudent to go easy on high-sodium processed foods to help keep your blood pressure normal and maybe prevent other serious health problems.

HERE'S WHAT YOU CAN DO

Whether you have high blood pressure, salt sensitivity, or just want to take measures now to prevent health problems from occurring, it's pretty clear that cutting back on sodium is good for all of us. The American Heart Association and American Diabetes Association recommend that we consume no more than 2,300 milligrams of sodium each day, which is right in line with the 2005 Dietary

Guidelines for Americans (the Institute of Medicine and the FDA recommend a sodium intake of no more than 2,400 milligrams per day and no more than 1,500 milligrams per day for people with hypertension). How much is 2,300 milligrams? It's about one teaspoon of salt. Most Americans consume at least twice as much, which is the equivalent of two or more teaspoons of salt. Some people need less than 2,300 milligrams per day, especially if they have kidney problems or congestive heart failure.

If you think you could stand to have a little less sodium in your diet, here are a few things to consider. First, remember that sodium is found in all of the foods that we eat. It's not wise or even possible to completely remove sodium from your diet (after all, it is an essential mineral). Second, keep in mind that the total amount of sodium you ingest in your daily diet is important, not just the sodium content of a specific food. This means that it's okay to occasionally eat a high-sodium food as long as the rest of your food intake is moderately low in sodium. Finally, the key to a healthy diet is to make gradual, small changes in your eating habits.

Rome wasn't built in a day, and it may not be feasible to stop eating all your favorite high-sodium foods overnight. If you're worried that foods will suddenly taste bland and dull, think about this: studies show that people who slowly reduced their sodium intake over time adapt to a low-sodium diet to the point that low-sodium foods taste good and high-sodium foods are too salty. By slowly making changes, you're less likely to notice any differences in how foods taste, and the changes you do make will be permanent ones.

1. **Shake the salt.** One quick and easy step you can take right now is to avoid adding salt to your foods, either in cooking or at the table. Start tasting your foods before automatically adding salt. You may be in the habit of reaching for the saltshaker before

eating, so try not to keep the saltshaker on the table or even near the stove. Do you automatically sprinkle salt into the pan of water when you cook rice or pasta? Try leaving it out next time; the water will still boil. You can also limit or even leave out the salt called for in most recipes. You'll never even miss it if you use other seasonings, such as black pepper, herbs, and spices. If you use packaged rice or pasta dishes, use only half of the seasoning packet. Doing this can save you up to 500 milligrams of sodium per serving. If you still feel you need to add some salt when cooking, add it toward the end, so the salt flavor won't cook away.

2. **Read nutrition labels on packages and containers of food.** The Nutrition Facts label on every packaged food must list the amount of sodium (in milligrams) contained in one serving of that food. Be sure to read the serving size because the amount listed as one serving may be a lot smaller than what you normally eat. In addition to the amount of sodium in one serving, the label will also show what percentage of the recommended daily value of sodium (2,400 milligrams) is provided in one serving. Keep in mind that a food labeled *Reduced Sodium, Unsalted,* or *No Salt Added* can still contain a significant amount of sodium. These claims do not necessarily mean that the food is low in sodium. Take a look at Chapter 8 to learn more about these terms and about how to read a Nutrition Facts label.

3. **Choose fresh, frozen, or canned foods without added salt.** Foods that are fresh or frozen (without salt added) are the best choices if you need to limit your sodium intake. Good examples are fresh fruits and vegetables; poultry, fish, and lean meats; and unprocessed whole-grain foods (breads, cere-

als, pasta, rice). If you use canned foods, buy those that are labeled with *No Salt Added* or empty the canned food into a colander and run it under water for a few minutes to rinse away some of the sodium in which it has been packed.

4. **Be careful when eating out.** If you eat out on a regular basis, you should be careful about your food choices in a restaurant. Many dishes can be very high in sodium. However, you can eat out and reduce your sodium intake by following a few simple guidelines:

   • Once again, ignore that saltshaker on the table.

   • Go easy on the condiments, such as mustard, catsup, soy sauce, and salad dressings, because they tend to be high-sodium foods.

   • Read menus carefully. Terms such as marinated, pickled, smoked, teriyaki, and "in broth" usually mean "high sodium."

   • Keep things simple. Foods that come with special sauces, gravies, or toppings are often high in sodium. If possible, order your foods plain. If you wish to try a sauce or topping, ask that it be served on the side.

   • Ask your server about any menu items for which you are uncertain of the sodium content. Also, request that your foods be prepared without added salt.

   • If you're eating at a fast-food restaurant, ask to see the nutrition information for their foods or look on the Internet for the nutrition information.

5. **Use salt substitutes with caution.** Many people switch over to salt substitutes as an alternative to the saltshaker. Most of these substitutes contain potassium instead of sodium. The downside with these is that they can often taste bitter. There is also a health concern: people with high blood

pressure who take medications that make the body retain potassium should check with their health care provider before using salt substitutes. These people can be at risk of retaining too much potassium in their bodies, which can lead to heartbeat irregularities. People with kidney problems need to heed this advice as well.

If you decide to use salt substitutes, keep in mind that some of them still contain sodium. It's important to read the label to be on the safe side. Remember, too, that you can always use seasoning products that have no sodium or potassium or make up your own mixture of herbs and spices to use in cooking and on foods.

6. **Check your medications.** Unfortunately, some medications may contain sodium. Examples are antacids, headache remedies, laxatives, and sedatives. If you need to take any of these medications, talk to your health care provider or pharmacist about lower-sodium alternatives.

SUMMARY

Having diabetes does not mean that you automatically have to cut salt and sodium from your diet. However, you do need to limit your sodium intake if you have high blood pressure; if you have prehypertension or are salt-sensitive; if you have congestive heart failure; or if you are prone to retaining fluid. What if you have none of the above? Well, it's still a good idea not to go overboard with the sodium, particularly if it means you can keep your blood pressure down and possibly *prevent* high blood pressure from ever developing. Plus, a low-sodium or moderately low–sodium diet may help keep your bones healthy. If you think you might benefit from a lower-sodium diet, speak with a registered dietitian who can help you tailor an eating plan that's both palatable and healthful.

YOUR TURN

Now it's your turn to recall some key points from this chapter. Let's see how you do!

1. You should limit your sodium intake to no more than _____ milligrams per day.

2. Most of the sodium in our diets comes from the saltshaker. True or false?

3. Soy sauce is considered a low-sodium condiment. True or false?

4. List three ways that you can decrease your sodium intake over the next month.

   _____

   _____

   _____

See APPENDIX A for the answers.

CHAPTER 12

SNACKS

> ## MYTH
>
> People with diabetes must eat a snack between meals and particularly at bedtime to prevent low blood glucose levels.

JOYCE: My doctor started me on some diabetes medications and wants me to lose about 25 pounds. I have been inactive lately because I injured my knee, and my weight just keeps going up and up. My friend told me I should eat snacks between meals and before bedtime to prevent my blood sugar from getting too low because of the diabetes medications. In the past two weeks, I actually gained four pounds. I feel like I will never be able to lose weight because I feel like I snack all day long. Can you help?

DIETITIAN: Don't worry, Joyce. Lots of people struggle with the decision of whether they should snack, regardless of whether they have diabetes or not. Snacking does have benefits and drawbacks; however, *smart snacking* is the key. Today, let's talk about your daily eating plan and activity level and when it may be best to eat a healthy snack and when you might want to choose not to eat a snack.

JOYCE: Does *smart snacking* mean only snacking when you feel a low blood sugar reaction coming on or when you are going to be exercising?

DIETITIAN: Actually, it means that if you are going to have a snack, it should be a planned, low-calorie, low-fat snack and not a snack that turns into another meal.

JOYCE: I know exactly what you mean. My dinner meal often goes on long after the meal is over. I snack until bedtime, and most of the time I end up feeling guilty and stuffed.

DIETITIAN: Well, today we can discuss why snacking can interfere with weight control and your ability to control your blood glucose level and how you can avoid snacking unless you are actually hungry or need food for exercise. We will also discuss why *planning* your snack food choices will keep you from overeating at meals.

WHAT'S NEXT

Like Joyce, many people with diabetes struggle with the issue of snacking. Joyce was receiving mixed messages about snacks. The first message was about weight loss: *if you want to lose weight, you have to cut down your calories and increase exercise.* The second message was about blood glucose control: *if you want to maintain control, you have to exercise, monitor your food intake, and snack between meals when blood sugar levels drop.* In her attempt to stay healthy, Joyce was trapped in a vicious cycle.

The dietitian helped Joyce understand that in order to maintain her weight, she must balance the calories she eats each day with the calories she burns for energy each day. When the calories are spread out over the whole day, within three meals and possibly some snacks, it is *still* only the total amount of calories eaten in the day that counts. Rather than eating consistent meals each day, Joyce often skipped meals in an attempt to save calories. Unfortunately, the saved calories in the earlier part of the day were quickly stolen for food eaten at the dinner meal that never seemed to end.

Together, Joyce and the dietitian devised an eating plan and also came up with a list of healthy smart snacks that were planned for *active* and *inactive* days. This plan, with three healthy meals a day, would help keep Joyce's appetite under control on inactive days and would provide adequate nutrients to keep her blood glucose stable between meals. On active days, snacks could be added to the three meals, depending on her activity level that day. Joyce also learned why certain types of snacks sustained (or carried) her appetite and maintained blood glucose better than others. Once Joyce understood how different foods affected her blood glucose, she was better able to eat healthily and exercise. She eventually dropped 25 pounds and was able to entirely stop taking her diabetes medications.

THE OLD AND THE NEW

Early in the 20th century, eating and sharing food was mostly a pleasant social experience. Unlike today, food and meals were not continually related to concerns about health, dieting, and weight. Not only were people able to enjoy the pleasures of the table, they were also better able to distinguish what a suitable portion looked like. They had not yet entered into the era of portion distortion.

At the start of the 20th century, America's eating habits were typified by a three-meal pattern. Most meals were eaten at home. Working adults and children usually came home for the noon meal. They took advantage of the daylight hours by rising at dawn to consume a very large breakfast meal of grains, starches, proteins, and fat to provide much needed energy for long hours of physical labor. They would then return home to eat their large, main meal at noon (dinner), only to return to more physical labor for the rest of the daylight hours. At the end of the day, they would eat what used to be known as the supper meal, which means a "light meal," before retiring for the night. Their meals were distributed throughout the daylight hours, and snacking was not the norm.

Toward the middle of the 20th century, new foods were offered in quantities meant to be eaten alone. The demand for convenient, ready-to-eat foods, which could be available in a short period of time, was on the rise. With the new food designs, we began developing new patterns of eating called *snacking*, meaning that food could be eaten at any time or place. Our eating patterns now included single-serving snack and convenience foods that were eaten between meals. These snack foods were initially converted from our country's staple foods, such as potatoes and corn, but gradually more and more calories from fats and sugars were added.

Now, at the beginning of the 21st century, the development, availability, and abundance of new foods in our country have caused us to lose much of the social aspect our food supply used to provide. We are often unable to truly enjoy the pleasures of the table, partly because of the many proven links that foods have to disease and weight. We know that food eaten in the company of family or friends definitely affects our nutritional status, and although we would like to maintain the social meaning of the daily three-meal pattern, many do not have the time to continue this practice. Prepackaged foods, fast food, take-out foods, and two-income families have diminished many of the pleasures of the table. We no longer have time to eat that big breakfast and noon meal. Skipping meals in the earlier part of the day and eating very large evening dinners and snacking at night have become the norm. Food is now only a break in our workday. These days, we eat less at home and snack more outside of the home. Only now are we learning more about the portion sizes that restaurants and take-out establishments offer, and they are often double what they should be.

As you can see below, people in the early 20th century ate a large breakfast, enjoyed a main meal (dinner) in the middle of the day, and ate the fewest calories at the evening meal (supper). Nevertheless, they regularly spaced out their meals over the day to enjoy the pleasures of the table.

Early in the 20th Century

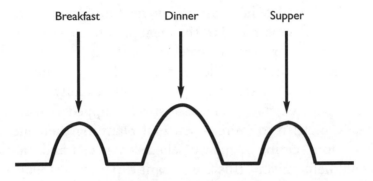

By the early 21st century, our main meal and the bulk of our calories have shifted toward the end of the day. We eat the smallest amount of calories during the day, overload on calories at the evening meal (what we call dinner), and then snack until bedtime.

Early in the 21st Century

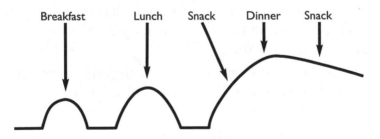

The way that we eat our meals is a good indication of what our blood glucose levels will look like. If we spread our food out over the day and do not skip meals, our blood glucose numbers will be more stable, or spread out, during the day.

HERE ARE THE FACTS

Because we tend to associate snacking with junk food, the shared public opinion is that snacking is harmful and unhealthy. However, whether you have diabetes or not, snacking can be an important part of your overall healthy eating plan, either every day or just on certain days.

For years, when people were started on insulin, snacks had to be added to the meal plan to cover the time when the older insulins would be peaking (that is, working their hardest) in order to prevent hypoglycemic (low blood glucose) reactions. Hypoglycemia usually occurred when people delayed a meal or snack, skipped a meal or a snack, or tried to exercise without planning their meals. Therefore, eating regularly scheduled meals and snacks could help prevent this unpleasant experience. Today, we have newer basal (or background) insulins that do not peak very much, and snacks are not forced on people with diabetes but can be eaten if needed.

People who are working toward weight loss may choose not to snack. Instead, they may make adjustments to their insulin doses or oral medications to avoid adding extra calories to their meal plan. It is really up to you if you want to include snacks in your diabetes meal plan. Check with your doctor or certified diabetes educator for help on how to do this.

There are many positive aspects that snacks can provide to help you control weight and blood glucose. Snacking can

- help prevent overeating at meals.
- provide a constant source of fuel to your body throughout the day.
- help trick the body into burning more calories, rather than storing them, by spreading your food throughout the day, so your body is never extremely hungry.

- regulate and improve blood glucose, because the body gets a frequent supply of fuel every three to four hours, rather than the typical feast-or-famine situation, in which you go from super hungry to super full.

WHAT SNACKING IS NOT

Snacking Is Not Grazing

Snacking is simply eating a small amount of food within a certain time frame, and it has a definite beginning and an end. Grazing means eating small amounts of food throughout the day. Although grazing may work for some, this method usually results in continuous binge eating and a free-for-all without a planned beginning and end.

Snacking Is Not Permission to Skip a Meal

Snacks should be planned and eaten between meals, not in place of meals. Proper snacking cuts down on real hunger, nibbling, and the risk of low blood glucose. If you try to avoid a snack or a meal to save calories and the result is low blood glucose, you will end up eating many more calories than if you had eaten the snack or meal in the first place. Skipping meals only deprives your body of fuel and allows your body to assume it has to conserve rather than burn calories.

Snacking Is Not Eating Junk Food

Although we tend to think about candy, cookies, and chips as typical snack foods, snacks are not meant to be empty-calorie foods. Empty-calorie foods are the invention of our country's food suppliers and simply do not furnish wholesome nutrition in spite of all the calories they add. Instead of allowing junk foods to take the place of more nutritious foods, try thinking of a nutritious snack as a mini-meal—that is, any food that you would include in a regular meal, but on a smaller scale.

Snacking Is Not a Cause of Weight Gain

Planned snacking between meals will only cause weight gain if you overeat at snack time. However, weight gain is often the result of not snacking. Here's why. Many Americans eat very little, if anything, at the breakfast meal. Later, if there is time, they have a quick lunch, and then end up eating a huge amount of calories while waiting for the dinner meal, at the dinner meal, and then continuously snacking until bedtime. So all of the calories saved during the day are quickly used up from 6:00 pm until bedtime. This common but harmful eating pattern denies your body of fuel in the early part of the day and provides too much fuel at the end of the day. This leads the fat cells to store away more calories, not burn them. When the food is spread out more evenly throughout the day, your body is better able to burn more calories efficiently.

Snacking Is Not Eating in Your Car, at Your Desk, or in Front of the TV

Snacking works best when you don't associate snack foods with too many different areas of your house and life, because these areas are likely to trigger a hunger reaction. When you eat a snack, try to sit down at a table and enjoy the snack, even if you only have five minutes to eat it. Remember, a very important thing to think about when considering snacking is location.

Snacking Is Not Keeping Junk Food in the House

For the most part, snacking is keeping your surroundings free of junk food. Only keep planned, healthy snacks in plain view at home or at work, with the intention of eating these snacks at consistent times each day and then be sure to *end* the snack. This does not mean that junk food can never be eaten, but save it for special occasions, such as when you are visiting friends, at office parties, eating out to celebrate a special event, or enjoying the holidays. Better yet, plan one or two days during the week when you will allow yourself one of your favorite junk foods as a snack. Buy that food only in single servings. That way, it is easier to plan the quantity so that you won't overeat. For instance, do not buy a large family-size bag of chips; buy a small, single-serving-size bag instead.

Snacking Is Not Being Hungry

Snacking allows an even flow of fuel (calories) to the body at planned intervals. This should allow most people to begin identifying the normal signals of hunger rather than unconsciously eating out of boredom or stress. We all need to become more aware of when, what, why, and where we are eating when it is not a specific mealtime, because following an erratic eating schedule prevents our bodies from signaling real hunger pangs.

HERE'S WHAT YOU CAN DO

Food suppliers have become more sensitive to our desire for more healthy snacks in our quest to remain healthy. Not only are we being provided with a variety of healthy snack choices, but these choices are also now available in single-serving sizes. Even cookies and chips are offered with less fat and calories, assuming that we only eat the indicated serving size and not the whole package. Below are some tips to help you turn your grazing into planned snacks and choose the best foods for smart snacking.

1. **Plan your snacks.** Visit with a registered dietitian to develop a meal plan that includes both meals and snacks and that will work with your home and work schedules. If your meal/snack schedule is written on a meal plan and in plain sight, it is more likely that your timing will become routine. When you know that your food

intake is planned, you will become less anxious while waiting for the next meal or snack.

2. **To get started, keep a written food record.** To better estimate when and where your snacking goes off track, keep a food record for one week, including the weekend. This record should include:

   When: the time of your meals and snacks

   What: the actual foods you eat and drink at meals and snacks

   How much: the amount of the foods eaten

   Why: the reason why you are eating (snack time, boredom, stressed)

   Where: the location when you are eating (car, desk, in front of TV)

   Keeping an honest food record will help you troubleshoot problem areas. This record will help you answer the following six questions:

   1. Is your food evenly spread out over the day?
   2. What interferes with your ability to eat consistent snacks?
   3. When and where do you tend to overeat?
   4. Are snacks helping you eat smaller meals?
   5. Have the snacks decreased large fluctuations in your blood glucose?
   6. Have you cut down the number of junk food snacks that you are eating?

3. **Choose long-lasting snacks.** A snack with staying power is usually a snack with carbohydrate combined with a small amount of lean protein and healthy fat. The list on p. 175 can be mixed and matched to meet your snack needs.

Commonly Asked Questions

When I have a craving for a special "treat" snack, what are some alternatives?

It is important to allow yourself some "treat" snacks once in a while, as long as you stay within your carbohydrate

One Carbohydrate	One Protein
The foods in this section each contain about 15 grams of carbohydrate (1 carbohydrate serving)	*The foods in this section each contain about 7 grams of protein (or 1 ounce)*
1 slice of whole-grain bread	1 ounce of low-fat cheese
1/2 whole-grain English muffin	1 Tbsp peanut butter
1 cup or 1 small piece of fresh fruit	1/4 cup low-fat ricotta cheese
1/2 of a 6-inch pita bread	1/3 cup hummus
2 plain rice cakes or popcorn cakes	1/4 cup low-fat cottage cheese
5–6 low-fat crackers	1 ounce of low-fat luncheon meat
5 pieces of melba toast	1 piece of light string cheese
3 cups low-fat popcorn	1 low-fat turkey or chicken dog
6 saltine crackers	1 hard-boiled egg
8 oz plain or 6 oz flavored light-style yogurt	1/4 cup nuts

allowance. Maybe you would like to spend your 15 grams of carbohydrate on a scoop (1/2 cup) of low-fat ice cream or frozen yogurt. How about a low-fat granola bar, a caramel popcorn cake, or 15 reduced-fat cheese puffs? Remember that all foods can fit as long as you make allowances in your daily plan.

How can I control bingeing on snack foods and not take in a lot of calories?

Select foods that can satisfy your hunger more quickly and sustain you for longer periods. If you feel a binge coming on, eat a few low-fat whole-grain crackers, a small piece of fruit, some raw vegetables, nuts, or seeds. Keep these fiber-rich foods stocked in your kitchen. They'll help fill you up and provide vitamins, minerals, and other healthful nutrients at the same time.

An appointment with a registered dietitian will help you determine what will work best for you. The dietitian will consider whether you need to snack by considering many factors, such as timing and types of meals, activity level, work schedule, medications (insulin or diabetes pills), your weight goals, and your actual hunger level due to the time between meals. A dietitian can also discuss with your doctor possible adjustments to your diabetes medications that will not require you to snack, if you so choose.

YOUR TURN

Now it's your turn to recall some key points from this chapter. Let's see how you do!

1. Snacks may also be added to your three meals on your meal plan when you plan to _____.

2. List three benefits of snacking:

   _____

   _____

   _____

3. List three things snacking is not:

   _____

   _____

   _____

4. Keeping written food records helps you determine when and where your snacking goes off track. True or false?

See APPENDIX A for the answers.

CHAPTER 13

EXERCISE

> ## MYTH
>
> People with diabetes should exercise every day in order to stay healthy.

ROBERT: I know exercise is important for me to stay at a healthy weight and to manage my blood glucose, but I'm having a hard time trying to fit in 90 minutes of exercise every day. I just don't have the time between work and family obligations.

DIETITIAN: It's a challenge for most people to fit activity or exercise in every day, given our busy schedules and lifestyles. Although regular exercise is important for good diabetes control, the good news is that you don't have to exercise every day to reap the benefits.

ROBERT: Well, I read somewhere that I should do some form of exercise every day, like walking or biking, and I get discouraged when I just don't have the time.

DIETITIAN: Fitting in *some* activity each day is ideal, whether you actually exercise, do some yard work, or even climb the stairs in your house or office building. Any activity that you do daily will help keep you fit, your heart and blood vessels healthy, and your blood glucose at a safe level. But doing some kind of aerobic activity at least three times a week is the goal.

ROBERT: I see. So if I walk or go to the gym at least three times a week, but do some activity every day, such as climbing stairs or doing yard work, I can be more fit, maintain my weight, and keep my diabetes in good control, too. That's definitely doable for me.

THE OLD AND THE NEW

Mention the word "exercise" and chances are, if you're like most people, you probably think of sore muscles, heavy breathing, and sweating…not to mention the difficulty of fitting it into your daily schedule. For many people, exercise brings back negative images of having to run around the track in grade school to sharing an aerobics class with spandex-clad twentysomethings while the instructor screams out orders like a drill sergeant. Or maybe you had an unpleasant experience during your last attempt at trying to get fit. Perhaps you went out and bought expensive running shoes and running clothes, then ran as fast as you could around the block, only to return home gasping for breath with a stitch in your side, barely able to walk the next day.

If this sounds familiar, don't despair. The meaning of exercise has greatly changed since grade school and even since the aerobic craze of the 1980s (remember "no pain, no gain"?). Would you believe that climbing a flight of stairs or two in your office, playing a game of Frisbee with your kids, gardening, or mopping the kitchen floor can give you some of the same benefits as jogging, biking, or skiing? No? Well, it can, and we're going to tell you how.

HERE ARE THE FACTS

Surprisingly, only 22% of adults in the U.S. are regularly active, meaning that they get some form of exercise at least three to four times per week. Yet, we all know that exercise is good for us. We've been hearing this for years. What many people may not know, however, is that 30 minutes of moderate exercise, such as walking or dancing, can be just as effective for disease prevention and overall good health as the same amount of time doing strenuous exercise, such as running. In other words, you don't need to sweat it out at the gym for 30 minutes or more every day, but you do need to try and accumulate at least 30 minutes of some kind of physical activity every day.

By the way, we sometimes use the words "exercise" and "physical activity" interchangeably, but they do have slightly different meanings. "Exercise" refers to specific activities that you do in order to become more fit. So, exercise includes jogging, using weights, taking an aerobics class, doing yoga, and more. "Physical activity" refers to any activities that you do to get your body moving, such as walking, climbing stairs, raking leaves, riding your bike, and vacuuming. Doing physical activity can help lower your blood glucose levels and make you feel better, both physically and mentally.

Benefits of Physical Activity for Diabetes

You may already have diabetes, but you may want to share the following information with family and friends, particularly if they are at risk of developing diabetes. Evidence from an important study called the Diabetes Prevention Program (DPP) has shown that active people are less likely to develop type 2 diabetes than inactive people. Many people who are at risk for developing diabetes also have high insulin levels in their blood, which can increase the risk of heart disease. Regular physical activity can help your body more efficiently use its insulin, as well. If you have type 2 diabetes, you know that your body has difficulty regulating the amount of glucose circulating in your bloodstream. Your cells may be insensitive to insulin, meaning that your insulin has trouble moving glucose into your cells to be used for energy. When levels of glucose stay high in the blood for long periods of time, diabetes complications can set in, such as kidney and nerve damage and eye problems. Weight loss is effective in lowering both blood glucose and blood insulin levels, but physical activity may be even more effective in increasing insulin sensitivity, thus lowering blood glucose levels and preventing or delaying diabetes-related complications.

If you already have diabetes, physical activity, along with a healthy eating plan, can help you better control your diabetes. You may even be fortunate enough to reduce the amount of diabetes medication (pills or insulin) you take or even get off your medications completely. (Never change the amount of your diabetes medication or stop taking your medication without discussing this with your doctor first.) The key is to make physical activity a regular part of your routine.

Benefits of Physical Activity for Weight Control

Physical activity is an important part of any weight reduction and maintenance program. It can supplement a reduced-calorie eating plan and help you achieve your weight loss goals. However, regular physical activity is probably most important for *maintaining* your weight loss. Physical activity alone, without reducing your calorie intake, only results in modest weight loss. In fact, the people who are the most successful in keeping their weight off have done so by following a program that combines healthy eating, regular activity, and behavior changes (such as not eating while watching TV).

Muscle is really the only tissue in the body that burns calories, because we use muscles to do almost everything, ranging from yawning or writing a letter to cross-country skiing. Muscles are constantly being broken down and rebuilt. Fat, on the other hand, is *much* less active than muscle. It burns hardly any calories. Fat deposits itself in fat cells and sits there until called upon as a reserve source of fuel. Our bodies easily accumulate fat and lose muscle if we're not physically active. This translates into a slower metabolism and, ultimately, weight gain. Even though you may be eating the same amount of food as you did in your twenties, it's possible that you'll gain weight as you get older due to your slowing metabolism. Physical activity helps you build and maintain muscle mass. The more muscle mass you have, the more calories you'll burn, even when you're relaxing. So, physical activity helps with weight loss and weight maintenance in two ways: by burning calories and by building muscle, which, in turn, burns calories.

HERE'S WHAT YOU CAN DO

It's never too late to become more physically active. You don't have to become a bodybuilder or go to the gym all the time. You will, however, need to fit some kind of physical activity into your schedule every day, along with doing both aerobic and muscle-strengthening exercises a few times a week to keep your metabolism burning steady while lowering your risk of diabetes complications. Here's what you will ultimately need to do:

> - At least 30 minutes of physical activity every day.
> - Aerobic exercise at least three times a week.
> - Strength training two to three times a week.

1. **Aerobic exercise.** Aerobic exercise helps get oxygen to your heart, which then helps get oxygen to your muscles. Your muscles can then use oxygen to produce energy. Aerobic exercise can burn anywhere from 200 to 400 calories every 30 minutes, depending on the type of exercise you are doing. For example, running will burn more calories in 30 minutes than walking for 30 minutes because the intensity of running is harder than walking. This doesn't mean, however, that you have to start running. Walking is an effective, safe, and easy exercise that will give you many of the same benefits as more strenuous forms of exercise.

   Other benefits of aerobic exercise are that it often helps reduce your appetite, so you consume fewer calories, and it helps keep your metabolism elevated for several hours after you stop exercising.

Some Examples of Aerobic Activities

walking	cross-country or
jogging	downhill skiing
jumping rope	playing sports, such as
swimming	basketball or tennis
dancing	mowing the lawn
ice skating	raking leaves
biking	

The goal is to do some type of aerobic exercise at least three times a week for at least 30 minutes. If you haven't been physically active for a long time, this can seem daunting. Don't worry. Start slowly and gradually. For example, you might start out walking around the block for 10 minutes. Then, walk for another 10 minutes later in the day. After you've mastered that, try walking for another 10 minutes after supper. Before you know it, you'll have done your 30 minutes of activity. It's okay if you break it up into shorter segments. As you get used to being active, every few days or every week, try adding on a minute at a time. You'll eventually find that you'll be able to walk 30 minutes at one time. If you find that you can't fit in 30 minutes on a particular day, then do what you can, even if it's fitting in a 10-minute walk at lunchtime.

If you choose to do something other than walking, such as housework or yard work, the intensity should be about the same as going for a brisk walk. How do you know if you're working out at the right level of intensity for you? A simple way to tell is to use the *talk test*, which measures the difficulty of your physical activity or exercise. When you take the talk test, you should be able to talk fairly easily while being active and not be gasping for breath. If you're gasping for air and can't speak, then ease up; you're working too hard. Conversely, if you can sing during your activity, you're not working out hard enough.

2. **Strength training.** Strength training prevents loss of muscle mass and helps build muscle mass. It's important to include some type of muscle-strengthening exercises in your routine to supplement your aerobic activities. Don't worry; you won't end up with bulging muscles if you don't want them. But you will have better muscle tone and more strength to help you perform everyday activities, such as carrying groceries or climbing stairs. Strength training can take the form of weight lifting (with dumbbells or barbells) or going to a health club and using the weight equipment. It can also come from doing calisthenics, such as sit-ups and leg lifts. You don't have to have a set of barbells, either. How about using cans of soup or plastic jugs filled with water? Whatever you choose to do to build lean body mass, you should aim for doing this at least twice a week, doing three sets of 8–10 repetitions (reps). However, you should not do the same strength training exercises every day. You need a day or two to rest between routines so your muscles can recover. If you're not sure how to get started, take a class at the local YMCA or YWCA or sign up for a few sessions with a certified trainer to make sure you stay safe and prevent injury.

Some people dismiss the idea of strength training because of health or medical problems or because they think they're too old to get started, but almost anyone can do some form of strength training. You must get your doctor's consent before starting any exercise program, but strength training can actually help increase bone mass, help people with arthritis move more freely, help prevent stiffness, help make you stronger, and help with weight loss. There's more: strength training can even help lower blood glucose levels and blood pressure, too. If you're an older adult, strength training can lessen the chances of you falling, helping you prevent injuries and maintain independence. Pretty amazing, isn't it?

3. **Getting started with exercise.** It's beyond the scope of this chapter to give you specific activities and training tips. If you've already increased your level of day-to-day physical activity (for example, walking for 30 minutes every day) and are ready to try something a little more strenuous, we recommend you consult with an exercise physiologist, preferably one who is also a certified diabetes educator (CDE). An exercise physiologist can prescribe an exercise program that is right for you and will take into account any health or medical problems you may have. This is very important, especially if you are considerably overweight or have high blood pressure, heart disease, arthritis, or diabetes-related complications such as neuropathy, retinopathy, or nephropathy. Don't assume the trainer at your local health club is qualified. He or she may not have the proper education and training. Ask your health care team about scheduling an appointment with an exercise physiologist if you have not been exercising and would like to start.

In addition to learning how to exercise safely and properly, it's important to discuss your plans with your doctor before you get started. Your doctor may recommend only certain types of exercise for you, especially if you have any medical complications. Specifically, notify your doctor before starting exercise if you:

- have high blood pressure
- have chest pain or have had a heart attack
- have irregular heartbeats
- have more than 20 pounds to lose
- are short of breath after mild exertion
- have wounds or cuts that don't seem to heal
- have pain in your calves, thighs, or buttocks when walking
- have retinopathy (eye disease)
- have neuropathy (nerve damage)
- have nephropathy (kidney damage)
- have uncontrolled blood glucose

Phew! That's a long list, we know. The good news is that even if you experience some of the above situations, you can most likely do *some* kind of exercise. Some forms of exercise are better than others for certain conditions. For example, people with retinopathy probably shouldn't do exercise that involves heavy weight lifting or straining. This doesn't mean that they can't use an exercise bike or a treadmill, though. If you have neuropathy in your feet or legs, you may not be able to walk very easily, but there are armchair exercises that you can most likely do instead. So you see, it's very important that you find out what is right for you.

COMMONLY ASKED QUESTIONS

I've heard that exercise can cause hypoglycemia. Is this true? What should I do about that?

If you're already physically active and take insulin or certain diabetes pills, you probably know by now that physical activity usually causes blood glucose to drop, sometimes to the point where it drops *too* low and you need to treat for a low blood glucose reaction. Remember that physical activity helps you use insulin more effectively, thus helping keep your blood glucose at a normal level.

Here's why you may experience hypoglycemia during exercise. If you exercise when your medication or insulin is peaking (that is, working its hardest to lower your glucose) and combine that with the increased effectiveness that physical activity gives to your insulin, then your blood glucose may drop too low (hypoglycemia). Hypoglycemia is defined as a blood glucose level less than 70 mg/dl. Common symptoms of hypoglycemia include feeling shaky, sweaty, lightheaded, irritable, or hungry. You might also have trouble concentrating or have a headache. Hypoglycemia can also occur if you haven't eaten enough beforehand, if it's been a few hours since your last meal or snack, or if you exercise longer or harder than usual. Other factors can play a role in causing hypoglycemia, such as the temperature, the humidity, and weather conditions (if you're outside). Remember, you may have a low blood glucose level during or after exercise. You may even have hypoglycemia *hours later*. This happens because your muscles are replenishing their stores of glucose by taking glucose from your bloodstream.

Always be sure to carry some form of fast-acting carbohydrate (such as glucose tablets, a tube of instant glucose gel, or a juice box) whenever you exercise, along with identification that shows that you have diabetes. You can limit your chances of having exercise-related hypoglycemia by doing a few things.

- **Adjust your insulin.** If you take insulin, talk to your health care team about adjusting your insulin, if necessary, to prevent lows. If your insulin is peaking during the time you plan to be physically active, this is the insulin that you'll likely need to adjust. For example, if you take a rapid-acting insulin and you plan to exercise after supper, you might need to decrease your supper dose by a few units. Your health care team can also help you adjust your insulin if you're going to be active for extended periods of time (when skiing or hiking, for example).

- **Adjust your medication.** If you take an oral diabetes medication, it is important that you *do not* make adjustments in the dosage without first discussing this with your health care team. However, you may find that with regular exercise and activity that you may be able to reduce your dose and maybe even eliminate the need for medication altogether. If so, bring this up with your health care team to see if you can make this change to your medication regimen.

- **Adjust your food intake.** There are times when you might need to eat a snack before exercising. It's a good idea to make some changes in your eating plan if *1*) your exercise or activity is unplanned and you've already taken your medication or insulin, *2*) you plan to exercise before a meal, *3*) you don't feel comfortable adjusting your insulin, or *4*) you expect to be strenuously exercising. For example, if you are exercising after a meal, you may want to increase your carbohydrate intake at that meal by 15–30 grams. Or, if you exercise between meals, it's a good idea to eat a snack of 15–30 grams of carbohydrate beforehand, such as a piece of fruit, a granola bar, or some peanut butter crackers. You must also take into account your blood glucose reading before you begin to exercise. Checking your blood glucose is crucial. Your dietitian or exercise physiologist can give you more food adjustment guidelines. If you're trying to lose weight, however, it's best to either learn to adjust your insulin or make sure that you choose healthy, low-fat snacks to keep your calorie intake under control. Also, if you take diabetes pills, ask your health care team if you're at risk for hypoglycemia, because not all pills cause low blood glucose. If you're on a pill that does not cause low blood glucose, you don't need to eat a snack before exercising. After all, you don't want to defeat the purpose of exercise by having to eat more.

Okay, what about hyperglycemia?

Believe it or not, exercise can actually have the reverse effect on your blood glucose—it can raise it. When you start to exercise, your liver releases glucose to make sure that your muscles have enough fuel, no matter what your blood glucose level may be. If you exercise when your blood glucose is on the high side, exercise can sometimes make your blood glucose go even higher. For people with type 1 diabetes, this can be a potentially dangerous situation. When you lack insulin and have high blood glucose, you can develop ketoacidosis, which is very serious and can be life threatening if it is not treated quickly.

If you have type 1 diabetes, we recommend that you not exercise when your blood glucose is 250 or higher and you have ketones in your urine or when your blood glucose level is above 300, with or without ketones. (Talk to your health care team if you're not sure how to check for ketones.) If you have type 2 diabetes, don't exercise if your blood glucose is 400 or higher.

How do I stay motivated to exercise?

People who don't exercise usually have a list of reasons describing why they can't. Often it's "I just don't have time" or "joining a health club is too expensive." Look past these excuses and what you'll see is a person who is perhaps afraid or hesitant about just getting out there and doing it. Most likely this person also feels guilty because he or she is *not* exercising and knows that he or she should. If you're one of these people, read the tips below. Maybe you'll change your mind after reading them!

- Consult with your health care provider to make sure it's safe for you to exercise. Then, try to meet with an exercise physiologist to develop a program that works for *you*, not for your neighbor.

- Wear comfortable workout clothes that fit. Also, invest in a good pair of sneakers that are appropriate for what you'll be doing.

- Don't do too much at once, even when the temptation is there. Start with 5 or 10 minutes if that's what you can comfortably finish. You'll quickly build up. Take it slow.

- Schedule an appointment for activity. Treat your exercise sessions just like your other appointments. Write them in your date book or on your calendar. By doing this, you're treating exercise as a priority.

- Enlist the support of family or friends. For example, if you're having trouble finding the time to exercise, maybe your spouse can take the kids to school a few mornings a week and you can exercise then.

- Do an activity, such as walking or taking a dance class, with a family member or a friend. That way, if you're not in the mood, your companion will be there to talk you out of skipping your workout.

- Do it alone. Some people find they do better when they are on their own. For them, exercise is a time to focus and reflect on the day or on important matters. Others find that exercising alone is more enjoyable than being in a class with other people and gives them much needed time for themselves.

- Do something you enjoy. If you hate using the exercise bike, you'll come up with 101 excuses not to use it. Ask yourself what you would like to do or, at least, what you'd tolerate doing. Perhaps walking or swimming appeals to you more.

- Still bored with the usual types of exercise? Try something new, like a spinning class, or tai chi. Or do something that you might not think of as exercise, such as swing dancing or country line dancing. Besides having fun and meeting new people, you'll get a great workout.

- Vary your routine. Walking the same route day in and day out can get boring. Try a new route or try a different activity altogether. Not only does this add variety, but because different exercises work different muscles, you'll end up with a more thorough exercise plan, too.

- Exercise to music. Upbeat, uplifting music often helps you soar through your workout, or try watching the news or your favorite TV show while you're exercising to help pass the time. Some types of exercise equipment, such as treadmills and stationary bikes, have room to attach a book rack. Now you can get smart and get fit at the same time.

- Set goals for yourself. If you're now exercising for 15 minutes a day, then make it your goal to work up to 20 minutes a day next week. When you reach your goals, reward yourself!

- Chart your progress. Just like you keep track of your blood glucose levels and your food intake, keep track of your exercise. This helps reinforce the importance of exercise and allows you to see how you're doing.

- Don't feel guilty if you can't fit in your usual walk or trip to the gym. Focus on making the most of whatever activity you are doing that day. After all, housecleaning, climbing stairs, raking, and gardening are all great ways to burn calories and get those chores done at the same time.

- Help others while helping yourself. If you've been walking or jogging for exercise, consider doing a race or walking or running for a good cause, such as the American Diabetes Association's annual Step Out to Fight Diabetes (formerly America's Walk for Diabetes).

YOUR TURN

Now it's your turn to recall some key points from this chapter. Let's see how you do!

1. List three benefits of exercise.

   _____

   _____

   _____

2. Hypoglycemia from exercise can be prevented by (circle all that apply):

         eating a snack before exercising

         taking more insulin

         taking less insulin

         drinking more water

3. It doesn't count unless you exercise for at least 30 minutes all at once. True or false?

4. List three things you will do to keep yourself motivated about exercise.

   _____

   _____

   _____

See APPENDIX A for the answers.

CHAPTER 14

DINING OUT WITH DIABETES

> ## MYTH
>
> People with diabetes shouldn't eat out.

JOANNE: I have to eat out for business at least four times a week, but whenever I do, my blood sugars go sky high! Then, hours later, it catches up with me, and I feel tired and sluggish.

DIETITIAN: It sounds like you're eating larger portions when you eat out or maybe you're not quite sure what to choose from the menu.

JOANNE: You know, I think you're right, because I've also gained about 10 pounds since starting my new job. The restaurants I tend to eat at seem to serve way more than I usually eat at home. Because I have to eat out so often, are there ways that I can eat out and still keep my weight and my diabetes under control?

DIETITIAN: Of course. It's not always easy, but there's no reason why you can't enjoy eating away from home and stay healthy at the same time. Let's talk about some healthier menu items that you can choose when you go out to eat.

JOANNE: That sounds great. I'm glad to hear that I can still eat out but make better choices.

What's Next?

These days, eating away from home seems to be more of a necessity than a treat. As Joanne is finding out, busy work or school schedules, power lunches, and frequent travel often make cooking and eating at home difficult. Plus, with the wide variety of restaurants available, eating out is fun, convenient, and quick. Besides, who wants to spend an hour cooking dinner after a long day at work?

The Old and the New

Back in the early 1950s, only about 25 cents out of every dollar spent on food was spent at a restaurant. Dining out was usually reserved for special occasions, such as birthdays and anniversaries. Today, eating out is still a treat for some of us, but it's an everyday thing for many of us, too. According to the *Consumer Expenditures in 2003* report of the U.S. Bureau of Labor Statistics, a household spends about $5,300 annually on food, and around 40% of that is spent eating away from the home. In fact, dining out is such big business that, in a 2006 press release, the National Restaurant Association claimed that restaurant sales were the "cornerstone of our nation's economy."

Another sign that times have changed is the size of dinner plates, both in restaurants and at home. Years ago, the average plate size was about eight or nine inches in diameter. Today, plates are several inches larger, averaging 12 inches. Studies show that people who eat from larger plates and bowls tend to eat larger amounts of food, which should surprise no one. So, obviously, restaurants tend to serve their meals on large plates because the more food they serve you, the more likely you'll come back.

Here Are the Facts

Compare restaurant meals with those you prepare at home. What you discover might surprise you. Restaurant portions are gargantuan. More than one course is served, starting with that basket of hot rolls and butter or tortilla chips and salsa. Most menu items are high in fat and calories, alcoholic beverages are often consumed before or with the meal, and the dessert menu beckons with its sinful offerings. Then, of course, there is the issue of timing of meals. In many cases, eating out means that you'll be eating later than usual, which can interfere with your diabetes medication schedule, particularly if you take certain diabetes pills. However, all is not lost. You can eat out and stay healthy at the same time. Believe it or not, it's possible to find healthful menu items in most restaurants and not stray too far from your eating plan while enjoying yourself at the same time.

Making Sense of Menus

Reading a menu can be a piece of cake if you know what to look for and what the various cooking terms mean. Most of us know that anything fried will also be high in fat, but what about *sautéed*, *parmigiana*, or *au gratin*? If you're able to navigate your way around a menu, it will be much easier for you to choose healthful items and steer clear of excess fat and calories. When in doubt, ask your server to explain whatever is unclear, whether it's the actual definition of a term or how a particular dish is prepared.

Go Ahead	Steer Clear
Baked (without butter)	Fried
Broiled (without butter)	Breaded
Roasted	Sautéed
Grilled	Creamed or creamy
Poached	Hollandaise
Steamed	Au gratin
Stir-fried	Scalloped/escalloped
Blackened	Buttered
Marinara	Alfredo
Cacciatore	Parmigiana
Au jus	Bearnaise

HERE'S WHAT YOU CAN DO

1. Refer to Your Meal Plan

Hopefully, by this point, you've met with a dietitian to establish some kind of an eating plan for yourself. (If you haven't, put this on your "to do" list.) This plan may involve using the Plate Method, traditional exchanges/choices, or carbohydrate counting. Whatever method you are using, make sure you have a sense of how many servings, exchanges/choices, or carbohydrate grams you need to aim for at that particular meal. Some people find that carrying a wallet-sized copy of their meal plan helps when eating out. Other people carry pocket-sized books that list carbohydrate and fat grams for various foods. There are even electronic versions of food lists that you can download to your PDA or cell phone.

2. Learn Serving Sizes

Okay, weighing and measuring foods isn't much fun. But you're not doomed to a lifetime of balancing a chicken breast on the scale or scooping pasta into a measuring cup. If you don't have a good sense of what a four-ounce piece of meat or one cup of mashed potatoes looks like, take a few minutes the next time you're cooking to measure or weigh out your portions. (One hint: always weigh and measure foods *after* cooking.) After you've measured your foods a few times, you will be able to more accurately estimate your portion sizes. Occasionally check your measuring skills to make sure those portions haven't all of a sudden doubled in volume.

Need some more help? Here's a trick you can use to gauge portions without having to lug your scale and measuring cups along to every restaurant you visit. Visualize these everyday items to help make things a little easier.

- A deck of playing cards = 3–4 ounces of protein
- A computer mouse = one medium potato
- A teacup = 1/2 cup ice cream or frozen yogurt
- A light bulb = 1/2 cup grapes
- A baseball = 1 cup fruit
- A tennis ball = one medium piece of fruit
- A walnut = 1 tablespoon of peanut butter

Another way to visualize portion sizes is to use your hands. Although everyone has differently sized hands, you can still use them to figure out how much food you think is on your plate. Here are some examples.

- The palm of your hand (without fingers) = 3–4 ounces protein
- A fist = 1 cup of pasta or 1 medium potato
- The tip of your thumb = 1 teaspoon of butter
- The length of your thumb = 1 ounce of cheese or meat or 1 tablespoon of salad dressing
- A cupped handful = 1–2 ounces of potato chips or pretzels (keep in mind that these handfuls are based on a woman's hand, so men need to eat a little less than this)

3. Plan Ahead

Planning ahead means several things. First, if you anticipate eating a meal with more fat one evening, be sure to eat less fat that day at breakfast and lunch. Or, if time permits, fit in some activity—such as a short walk around the block after your meal—to burn off some of those calories and keep your blood glucose levels under better control. Second, don't skip lunch or your afternoon snack (if you eat one) to save room for dinner. You'll be too hungry by the time your meal is served and will likely end up eating too much. Plus, if you take certain diabetes pills or insulin and don't eat enough earlier in the day, you may end up with low blood glucose. Third, call the restaurant ahead of time to inquire about the types of meals served and to ask if food can be prepared with less fat or sodium, for example. Some restaurants make their menus available online so that you can decide what you'll order before you even go to the restaurant.

4. Take Home Leftovers

With the size of restaurant meals these days, it's no wonder people end up leaving the restaurant groaning and loosening their belts. Don't feel compelled to clean your plate of every morsel. Why not eat a reasonable portion, take the rest home, and have another meal the next day? Whether you call this "doggy-bagging" or bringing home leftovers, most restaurants will happily accommodate your request to package up whatever you don't eat.

If you're a lifelong member of the "Clean Plate Club," cancel your membership and ask your server to pack up half your meal in the kitchen before it's served to you. By doing this, you can avoid overeating and you've got food for tomorrow's lunch or supper. Don't force yourself to eat everything on your plate.

5. Share a Meal

Restaurant meals tend to be big enough for two people, so why not split a meal with your spouse or friend? If you like, order a salad, an extra potato or serving of rice, and maybe an extra vegetable. That should be plenty for everyone. Now, what about dessert? Once again, consider ordering one order of tiramisu or pie for the table and having just a taste. Everyone will probably appreciate the calories saved and still enjoy that decadent dessert. Anyway, it's always the first bite that tastes best.

6. Ask!

Be assertive with the server and politely, but firmly, let them know how you would like your entree prepared. For example, ask how many ounces the salmon weighs (remember, restaurants give the weight of meat, poultry, and fish before they're cooked—these foods lose about

25% of their weight after cooking), for the dressing to be served on the side, or for your scallops to be broiled without butter. Many restaurants have fresh fruit, low-fat salad dressings, and sugar-free syrups available, although these items may not be listed on the menu. Ask for substitutions, too. Instead of the French fries, ask for more vegetables. Don't be afraid to speak up. You don't have to let anyone know that you have diabetes, either. More and more people are eating healthfully for many reasons, not just diabetes, and restaurants are used to such requests. Remember that restaurants are service-oriented establishments and they pride themselves not only on the quality of their food, but also on how well you are served. After all, they want you to come back.

7. Banish the Breadbasket

A warm basket of freshly baked rolls or loaf of bread can hit the spot while you're waiting for your meal to be served. However, they may be so good that you can't stop at just one. If you like, help yourself to that roll, but then ask your server to take the basket away. Another suggestion is to order a bowl of broth-type soup or a tall glass of seltzer water to sip on, which will help fill you up and keep you from reaching for another piece of bread.

8. Order from the Appetizer Menu

If you're looking for a light meal, check out the appetizer section of the menu. You may be able to make a meal of two or three appetizers and bypass the heavier entrees. Good choices can be shrimp cocktail, steamed clams, broth-based or tomato-based soups, raw vegetables, and small salads. To round off the rest of your meal, order a baked potato, rice, or extra vegetables a la carte (or individually). Just be sure to skip the fattier appetizers, such as nachos, mozzarella sticks, and buffalo wings.

9. Beware the Buffets!

Buffets and all-you-can-eat-style restaurants can spell disaster for many diners. After all, who doesn't want to get his or her money's worth of food? Before you dig in, walk around the buffet to see what is offered. Look for the food items that are lower in fat, such as vegetables, salads, poultry, and fish, and plan your meal around these items. For a treat, try one or two dishes that you don't usually eat. Don't feel like you have to heap food on your plate, either. You can always go back to try something else. Try not to let these situations throw you off your eating plan. If you have a hard time controlling yourself at buffet-style restaurants, try to limit how often you eat at them.

10. Go Easy with Alcohol

Many of us enjoy having a drink or glass of wine with our meals as a way to relax at the end of a busy day. However, the temptation to overindulge with good food and alcohol is frequently present. People with diabetes need to be careful when drinking alcoholic beverages and must understand how alcohol can affect diabetes control. First, realize that alcohol is a drug, just like your diabetes medication or aspirin. All drugs must pass through the liver to be detoxified and broken down. If you drink more alcohol than your liver can handle, then the alcohol can affect your central nervous system and lead to the symptoms of intoxication (what we normally call being "tipsy" or "drunk"). Second, if you take insulin or certain diabetes medications, you may be at risk for low blood glucose (hypoglycemia). Although most people with diabetes can drink alcohol in moderation, if your blood glucose levels are not well managed or if you have just finished a game of vigorous tennis or some other kind of physical activity, drinking alcohol can set you up for potentially severe hypoglycemia. The risk for hypoglycemia after having just one or two drinks is higher, especially if you have not eaten for a while.

Use common sense if you decide to drink. Don't drink alcohol if you are pregnant; have a history of alcohol abuse; have heart, liver, or kidney disease; have high triglyceride (blood fat) levels; or have poorly controlled diabetes. Always eat something that contains carbohydrate when drinking alcohol. Ideally, have the drink with your meal. If you're at a party and haven't had supper yet, make sure you have a few crackers or pretzels. Don't substitute alcohol for carbohydrate choices in your meal plan. If you're concerned about the calories in alcoholic drinks, substitute one drink (12 ounces of beer, 5 ounces of wine, or 1 1/2 ounces of liquor) for two fat choices. If you take insulin before your meal, it's best not to count alcohol as carbohydrate (even though many alcoholic beverages do contain carbohydrate) until you learn how certain alcoholic beverages affect your blood glucose levels.

11. Deal with Delays

Frequently, eating out means that meals may be served later than when you usually eat. If you take diabetes medications that don't work to directly lower your blood glucose, a delayed meal is not much of a concern. However, some diabetes medications, such as glyburide, glimepiride, and glipizide, can lower your blood glucose too much if you don't eat around the same times every day.

If you take insulin, you also need to be aware of when your insulin is peaking and when you'll be eating. If you take rapid-acting insulin before meals, it's easier and safer if you bring your insulin with you to the restaurant. This way, you don't have to worry about hypoglycemia while you're waiting to be seated or for your meal to be served. Talk to your health care provider about how to best deal with delayed meals.

12. Rethink Your Strategy

Eating out often seems like a necessity, because it's convenient and enjoyable. But if you're running into issues with your diabetes control (and your weight), you might consider eating out less often. Try bringing lunch to work a few times a week or cook a few meals ahead of time for the week ahead.

COMMONLY ASKED QUESTIONS

I have to eat out at least three times a week because of my schedule. How can I control my portions?

First, make sure you meet with a dietitian to work out a meal plan. Then, practice portion control at home, using measuring cups, spoons, and a scale. These tools will help you train your eyes to identify portion sizes when you're eating out. Also, try out the Plate Method. Aim for one-half of your plate to be filled with low-carbohydrate vegetables, such as broccoli, spinach, or carrots. Fill a quarter with a carbohydrate food such as a small potato or a serving of brown rice. Fill the last quarter of your plate with protein, such as fish, chicken, or lean meat. Finally, remember that it's okay to leave food on your plate. Take your leftovers home for another meal the next day.

If I drink a glass of beer, don't I have to substitute it for the carbohydrate at my meal?

No, the beer is in addition to your meal. Alcohol lowers blood glucose levels, so don't eliminate your carbohydrate food at a meal. If you take certain diabetes pills or insulin and don't eat some carbohydrate at your meal, then you might end up with a low blood glucose level later on. If you're concerned about the calories from beer, choose a light beer and eat less fat at your meal.

Sometimes the restaurant is slow at serving my meal, but I've already taken my insulin. I'm concerned about hypoglycemia. What can I do?

When you eat out next, take your insulin when your meal is right in front of you. However, this will require that you bring your insulin to the restaurant with you, so you might want to ask your health care team about using an insulin pen. An insulin pen is an easy, convenient, and discreet way to take insulin; you don't need to worry about vials and syringes.

Thinking that any seafood dish is low in fat, I ordered broiled scallops the other evening at a restaurant. When it was served, it was swimming in butter! What should I do next time?

Don't always assume that broiled or baked foods are low in fat. The best thing to do is to ask your server how a dish is prepared before you order. If it sounds like too much fat is used in the cooking process, ask if the kitchen can prepare your dish with less fat or at least a healthier fat, such as olive oil.

Sometimes I end up overeating when I go out to eat. Is it okay to take a little more insulin after my meal to prevent my blood glucose from going too high?

If you end up eating more than what you planned, it's okay to take insulin after your meal, but only if you know how much insulin to take for the extra carbohydrate you've just eaten. If you take a fixed dose of insulin or use a sliding scale, it's best not to take more insulin after eating because this could lead to hypoglycemia later on. If you've overindulged at a meal, the best advice is to get some physical activity after you've eaten (go for a walk, do some housework, or hop on the exercise bike). This will help lower your blood glucose and burn calories at the same time. At the next meal, get back on track with your usual eating plan.

Your Turn

Now it's your turn to recall some key points from this chapter. Let's see how you do!

1. List three things you can to do to eat more healthfully when eating out.

   _____

   _____

   _____

2. Drinking alcohol on an empty stomach can lead to high blood glucose levels later. True or false?

3. Which way is seafood best ordered: sautéed, grilled, or fried?

4. Measuring your foods at home can help you better recognize and measure portions at a restaurant. True or false?

See APPENDIX A for the answers.

CHAPTER 15

DIABETES AND FOOD CRAVINGS

MYTH

People with diabetes don't get food cravings.

SARAH: I generally do well with my eating plan, but every now and then I just crave something sweet. I simply break down and end up eating a whole box of cookies or anything chocolate. I can't control it! Then later on, my blood sugars are sky high, of course.

DIETITIAN: What brings on these cravings? The time of day? Stress? Do you think you're maybe depriving yourself of the foods you really like?

SARAH: Now that you mention it, I think most of my cravings tend to happen mid-afternoon at work, particularly when I'm feeling a little stressed out and tired. Sometimes at night I find myself eating ice cream right out of the container when I'm upset or anxious about something.

DIETITIAN: You're not alone. Everyone experiences food cravings at some time or another. The key is to learn how to deal with them before those cravings (and your blood glucose levels) get out of control. Why don't we look at some ways that might help you control those cravings and your blood glucose levels, too.

What's Next?

Does Sarah's plight sound familiar? A craving is defined as a consuming desire, longing, or yearning for something. We all have cravings at some point or another in our lives, whether it's for food, money, or companionship, but understanding and dealing with food cravings is complex. There are many theories and ideas as to why people experience these cravings, and yet there's not much agreement as to why they occur. What we do know about these mysterious and often frustrating cravings is that they happen because of a combination of physical and psychological factors. In other words, some of these may be in your head, so to speak, but some arise because of hormonal changes in the body. Let's take a look at this intriguing aspect of nutrition.

The Old and the New

Do Our Bodies Know Best?

The idea that the body craves the nutrients that it is lacking dates back to the early part of the 20th century. In the late 1920s, a pediatrician named Clara Davis published results of a study she conducted. In this study, three infants, aged 7–9 months old, were offered a variety of healthy foods from which to choose. All on their own, the infants chose foods that comprised a healthy diet, almost as if by instinct. Years later, in 1940, a psychologist named Curt P. Richter published a study of a young boy who obsessively craved salt, often eating it straight from the saltshaker. When this boy was hospitalized and denied salt, he died. This boy had an adrenal gland disorder that caused his body to lose salt. The boy was eating salt to keep him alive.

In more recent years, research by Judith Wurtman, a nutritional biochemist at the Massachusetts Institute of Technology, has provided more evidence that our bodies often give us signals when something is wrong with our diets. Dr. Wurtman has specifically studied people who are called "carbohydrate cravers." These people feel more energetic and less depressed after they eat carbohydrate-rich foods, such as bread or pasta. In fact, Dr. Wurtman has noticed that carbohydrate cravers are more likely to suffer from seasonal affective disorder (SAD), which is when people become more listless and depressed during the dark winter months. Eating carbohydrate-rich foods during this time of the year helps people who suffer from SAD feel better. This mood improvement likely has something to do with the release of a brain chemical called serotonin. Serotonin has a calming effect in the body. Dr. Wurtman's research lends weight to the idea that by craving carbohydrates, the body is attempting to correct an imbalance or deficiency.

Can Chemicals Cause Cravings?

Judith Wurtman's theory on carbohydrate cravers enters into the realm of how brain chemicals influence not only how we eat and why we eat, but also our thoughts, feelings, and moods. The brain produces many substances, called neurochemicals, which can affect our appetite and influence our food choices. Serotonin is one such neurochemical, called a neurotransmitter, which is produced from the amino acid tryptophan. Eating carbohydrate-containing foods triggers the entry of tryptophan into the brain, where it's used to form serotonin. Serotonin, in turn, has a calming, relaxing effect. The carbohydrate-serotonin theory suggests that an inadequate amount of carbohydrate in the diet causes serotonin levels to drop, leading to cravings for carbohydrate-rich foods, especially cakes, candies, and other sweets.

Not everyone fully agrees with this theory. Some researchers believe that people tend to crave fat rather than carbohydrate. Have you ever noticed what foods you eat when you have a craving? Chances are, if you have a sweet tooth, you'll eat "sweet fats," such as ice cream, cookies, or chocolate, instead of bread, crackers, or fat-free ice cream. So, the thinking is that it may be the fat in these foods that we really want and the added sugar just makes that food taste even better. The combination of fat and sugar releases endorphins in the brain, which are opiate-like chemicals that lift your mood and create an intense feeling of pleasure. Endorphins also act like the body's own natural painkillers. No wonder we find a piece of fudge or chocolate chip cookies more satisfying than a carrot stick!

Serotonin isn't the only neurochemical that plays a role in food cravings and appetite control. Another neurochemical, neuropeptide Y (NPY), may actually trigger the desire for carbohydrates. NPY is released when the body is depleted of carbohydrates, such as after strenuous exercise or a period of fasting. The inclination is to eat carbohydrate-rich foods in these situations, probably because of NPY. Galanin, another neurotransmitter, triggers the urge to eat high-fat foods, such as red meats, rich desserts, and creamy pasta sauces. Galanin levels tend to rise as the day goes on, when estrogen levels are high, and during weight loss. There is some evidence that obese people may have higher galanin levels than people of normal weight, which means that too much galanin or NPY secretion may eventually lead to weight gain. More recent research points to a link between food cravings, gambling, and drug addiction. Two hormones, called ghrelin and leptin, help control hunger and satiation (fullness) signals in the brain. Ghrelin, which is made in the stomach, triggers feelings of hunger. Leptin, however, signals the brain to stop eating and burn more fat. These two hormones apparently are also involved in the desire that typifies drug addictions, such as to cocaine. This research may eventually lead to treatment for food cravings and addictive behaviors.

Not surprisingly, stress plays a big role in food cravings. Remember Sarah and how she eats when she feels stressed? When we are under stress, our bodies release stress hormones, including cortisol, epinephrine, and norepinephrine. Although epinephrine and norepinephrine can increase heart rate and blood pressure, it's cortisol that has recently received so much attention due to its links with stress and an increase in unhealthy abdominal fat. Chronic stress raises levels of cortisol in the body, which can lead to weight gain, as well as more serious problems, such as depression, diabetes, and heart disease. High levels of cortisol can trigger pleasure-seeking behaviors, such as overeating, as a way to help handle stress. In fact, it's typical for people to crave comfort foods (such as bread, chocolate, mashed potatoes) during times of stress. Because most comfort foods aren't low in calories or fat, a person who is constantly stressed out may compensate by eating too much and thus gain weight. Unfortunately, dieting to lose any weight gained can actually backfire. Low-calorie diets can leave one feeling hungry, and the process of losing weight is perceived by the body as being stressful. In turn, more stress hormones are released, leading to a vicious cycle. This biochemical process is even more frustrating if you have diabetes and are struggling to control your blood glucose.

HERE ARE THE FACTS

As you can see, the science behind food cravings is complex. Food cravings often occur when you change your eating habits and start restricting or cutting out the foods that you like. For example, if you were told you could never eat a chocolate chip cookie again, what do you think you'd want all of a sudden? It's simple: the cookie.

Obviously, some people with diabetes do frequently feel this way. Most people with diabetes are given a meal plan or some kind of nutrition guidelines to follow for blood glucose control. A meal plan, while helpful and effective, pretty much tells you what you can eat, how much you can eat, and when you can eat. Spontaneous eating seems out of the question. If you're hungry at 5:00 p.m. but supper isn't supposed to be until 6:00 p.m., when you take your diabetes medication, what are your choices? You can wait it out, but more often than not, you end up grabbing a handful of crackers or chips and feel guilty a little while later.

People who follow strict weight loss plans often experience food cravings, too, and it's no wonder why: they get hungry! How long can a meal of baked chicken and steamed broccoli with fat-free margarine satisfy you? Think back to your previous weight loss attempts. Did you ever try one of those diets where you ate just one or two foods for days at a time? How long did that last? Probably not too long. You were probably counting the minutes until you could have a slice of pizza or cake. Restrictive diets are not only potentially unhealthy, but they're also one of the worse culprits for triggering food cravings and can lead people to overeating and bingeing (both of which can send your blood glucose levels out of whack).

Fortunately, we're learning more about food cravings all the time, and although they may always partly remain a mystery, we're much closer to understanding why they occur. We also have learned about effective ways to deal with them. The good news is that it is possible to occasionally enjoy your favorite foods while still controlling your diabetes and waistline at the same time.

The Cravings-Diabetes Connection

If you have diabetes, you already know that meal planning plays an important role in your diabetes management. Maybe you haven't thought much about this, except to notice that you need to eat meals on time, read food labels, and count carbohydrate grams. Did you ever stop and realize how much time you spend thinking about food? Diabetes can do this. Dietitians often hear people new to diabetes say, "I never used to eat candy before my diabetes, but now that's all I crave." Another typical complaint often heard by dietitians is that people with diabetes who need to eat meals and snacks on time spend the day constantly thinking about food, to the point that they almost become obsessed.

Dieting, whether it is for weight reduction or blood glucose control, imposes its own rules and regulations on you. In a sense, you no longer have control over what, when, and how much you eat. It should come as no surprise, then, that you may not be pleased with the idea of dieting over the long term, and you're not alone. On top of following a diet, you're also told that you must regularly check your blood glucose levels, take your medication as directed, exercise, get your eyes examined yearly, and so forth. The list is long. When you can't and don't live up to all these expectations, you may either feel guilty or adopt a devil-may-care attitude because you can't be perfect 100% of the time. Many people give up and end up bingeing on foods that aren't on the meal plan.

If you can identify with some of these concepts and are feeling confused or trapped, it's important that you talk to your health care team. If you're experiencing feelings of deprivation in regard to food, work with a dietitian who can show you how to fit those favorite foods into your eating plan without throwing off your blood glucose levels. In addition, it's particularly important to find a dietitian who will teach you that no foods are all "good" or "bad"—any food can fit into a healthy eating plan. If you take insulin, talk to your health care team about learning how to adjust your insulin for the occasional extra carbohydrate you'd like to eat.

Make sure that you monitor your blood glucose, especially when you splurge or try foods that you haven't eaten for a while. Check your blood glucose before you eat a meal and about two hours later to see how that particular food has affected your blood glucose. Keep a record of your results and show them to your health care team, especially if your results are high. They can help you think of ways to prevent high blood glucose after eating, whether through adjusting diabetes medication or insulin or increasing physical activity. Yes, you can have your cake and eat it, too!

Taming Your Cravings

While you'll probably never be able to banish your food cravings completely, there are ways to help you manage those cravings before they result in something more drastic, such as an eating binge. As we mentioned earlier, people with diabetes can be prone to eating challenges, depending on the advice they've been given by their health care team. After all, if your doctor has told you to never eat brownies again, then you can be sure that brownies will be a constant visitor in your nightly dreams.

In some instances, maybe you've been too hard on yourself in an effort to improve your blood glucose levels. Some people, after learning they have diabetes, develop their own a list of forbidden foods and their own particular way of eating. Unless you're used to rigidity and discipline, chances are you'll have difficulty following this way of eating for long. Instead, learn how to eat healthfully by getting help from your dietitian. Don't deprive yourself of the foods that you love, either.

Let's discuss some techniques that may prove useful to you. The first step is to learn the difference between *hunger* and *appetite*. Surprisingly, many people have no idea what it feels like to experience true physical hunger, whose indicators include stomach rumbles, hunger pangs, and headaches. People with diabetes are usually told that they have to eat at regular times each day, whether they feel hungry or not; therefore, they can lose sense of what being hungry actually feels like. Appetite, on the other hand, differs from hunger in that it can be triggered by certain emotions, places, smells, or events (think of your mother's homemade stuffing on Thanksgiving). Hunger is more physiological (or having to do with the body), whereas appetite is more psychological (having to do with the mind).

If you're not sure how to tell one from the other, you're not alone. It may take some practice, but the next time you experience a food craving, ask yourself the following questions. (Remember, it's okay to give yourself permission to feel hungry once in a while—in fact, it's a good thing to do this—as long as your blood glucose control isn't affected.)

- **When was the last time I ate?** If it's been more than four hours since you last ate, chances are that your stomach is empty and it's signaling you to eat something to keep your body fueled.

- **Am I feeling hunger or my appetite?** Again, if it's been a while since you last ate, you feel a little lightheaded, or your stomach is growling loudly, it's probably hunger. However, if you ate lunch an hour ago but someone in your office brought in a batch of homemade brownies and the smell is wafting into your cubicle, say hello to your appetite. The smell of something delicious can trigger your appetite, fooling your brain into feeling hungry, even when you're not.

- **Why do I want to eat right now?** Did you have a fight with your spouse or a bad day at work? Are you bored or feeling lonely? Emotions are strong triggers for eating, especially uncontrollable eating. Take a few moments to think about your feelings.

- **What am I craving?** Whether you truly feel hunger or your appetite has been stimulated by a certain event or place, it's important to identify what it is you want. You may be surprised to find that what you really want is to soak in a nice, hot bath or to talk to a good friend on the phone.

Here's What You Can Do

Now that you can distinguish between hunger and appetite, you're ready to tackle those cravings head on. Cravings will never go away for good, but you can take some measures to make sure they don't get out of control.

1. Know Your Emotional Triggers

As we mentioned earlier, emotions can be powerful triggers of eating. Stress, boredom, and loneliness can often lead to eating, especially those comfort foods that soothe us, at least initially. The problem, of course, with constantly eating to deal with emotions (or "feeding your feelings") is that not only do you end up consuming far more calories than you need, but you also don't solve the problem. Instead of reaching for that package of cookies the next time you feel stressed, try some of these activities:

- treat yourself to a massage
- go for a walk
- call a friend
- write a letter
- drink a cup of hot tea
- take a long, relaxing bath
- take up a hobby, such as knitting or wood carving

In fact, why not make a list of your own? That way, when emotions strike, you'll have an action plan ready so you can deal with your situation. If, despite all your efforts, your emotions constantly seem to get the better of you, then it may be wise to discuss this with your health care team. They may recommend that you get professional help.

2. Know Your Environmental Triggers

Your environment also plays a role in what, when, and how much you eat. For example, going to a party often leads to overindulging, simply because you're having fun.

Are you a sports fan? If you went to any baseball or football games this past season, did you eat your share of hot dogs and peanuts? Sometimes your home environment can be the culprit. It's all too common for people to sit down to watch TV after a hard day at work and end up mindlessly snacking throughout the night. This can be a particularly tough habit to break, but it's not impossible. Here are some tips to help you break the TV-eating connection:

- avoid keeping fatty, tempting goodies in the house
- ask family members to keep treats out of your sight
- eat only in one room: the kitchen or dining room
- drink water, sugar-free beverages, or hot tea
- have raw vegetables handy for a low-calorie snack

Another helpful piece of advice is to keep a food journal. Write down everything you eat and drink and why. After a few days, you may see a trend emerging. At this point, think of an action plan to counteract the pattern.

3. Wait Out Those Cravings

Cravings can vary in intensity. They may gradually build up, peak in intensity, and then fade away, almost like waves in the ocean. If you realize that cravings will come and go, you can prepare yourself. The next time an urge hits you, try waiting about 20 minutes for it to subside. Distract yourself by doing some chores, paying bills, or talking to someone. You may be pleasantly surprised that the craving has gone away.

4. Get Going!

Exercise can take your mind off eating and may help suppress your appetite. In addition, studies show that aerobic exercise, such as walking or riding a bike, can stimulate the release of endorphins, chemicals in the brain that relieve pain and make us feel good.

5. Separate Eating from Other Events

All too often, eating is combined with watching TV, reading, or doing work at your desk. The process of eating should be treated as its own event. In other words, do nothing else when eating. You'll enjoy it more, and you may be surprised that you end up eating a lot less. In fact, studies show that people who sit down at a table and focus just on their eating end up eating more slowly and eating less. At the same time, the craving for high-fat snacks may subside once you limit eating in front of the TV.

6. Drink, Drink, and Drink More

Nutrition experts all agree that an easy, effective way to curb cravings is to drink plenty of water. Liquids take up space in your stomach and give the appetite center in your brain the message that you're full. Although there's no magic amount of fluid to aim for each day, it's not a bad idea to drink least 8–10 glasses of water or other non-caloric fluids every day. By the way, some scientists think that it's best to avoid filling up on too many sugar-free beverages, such as diet soda or sugar-free lemonade. These scientists suggest that even though these drinks contain non-caloric sweeteners, their sweet taste may actually intensify your craving for sweet foods. If you think this might apply to you, shy away from sweet drinks and stick with water. Flavor it with lemon or lime for variety. You might even try sipping on hot tea or clear broth. Some studies have shown that people who drink hot liquids eat less.

7. Eat Regular Meals and Snacks

Okay, we said earlier that you should only eat when you feel hungry. But some people go all day without eating and end up with unbearable cravings and munchies at night. It's still important to eat at least three meals a day, with snacks between, if necessary. Some people do even better with six small meals each day. Eating several small meals every day may help your blood glucose management, reduce the number of cravings you get, and prevent overeating at night.

8. Fit in Fiber

Fiber is an indigestible carbohydrate that has no nutritional value (see Chapter 3) but does help increase satiety (fullness). Just think how you feel after eating a bowl of bran cereal for breakfast. Foods that are high in fiber include whole-grain breads, cereals, crackers, fruits, and vegetables. These foods take a while to chew and therefore slow down your eating rate, and they also take up room in your stomach, making you feel full sooner.

9. Turn Up the Heat!

If you like hot, spicy foods, such as Mexican, Thai, or Szechuan dishes, go ahead and indulge. Spicy foods tend to satisfy your taste buds quicker than bland foods, so you usually eat less. You can put some heat in your dishes at home by adding chili powder, jalapeno peppers, or horseradish. Spicy foods can also speed up your metabolism.

10. Count Carbohydrates

People who get at least 40% of their daily calories from primarily low glycemic index carbohydrate foods, such as oatmeal, brown rice, and sweet potatoes, tend to have fewer cravings for sweet carbohydrate foods, such as cookies and candy. Foods with a low glycemic index break down into glucose more slowly and don't lead to a rise in blood glucose levels as quickly as foods with a higher glycemic index. Keep in mind that not all foods with a low glycemic index are healthy choices, and remember that carbohydrate is the nutrient that has the most impact on blood glucose levels; therefore, people with diabetes need to control their total carbohydrate intake. This does not mean, however, that you should be on a low-carbohydrate diet. Instead, keeping your carbohydrate intake consistent on a daily basis will help you maintain blood glucose levels and keep those cravings at bay. Try to limit your intake of sugary carbohydrates, too. They contain empty calories and can trigger cravings. If you're not already doing so, talk with your dietitian about learning how to count carbohydrates in your eating plan and learn about the glycemic index. For more information on carbohydrate, see Chapters 2 and 3.

11. Go Ahead and Give In

What? You mean it's okay to indulge that craving? That's right. It's important not to completely deny yourself of the foods you love. Every now and then, especially when all other measures have failed, indulge a little and let yourself enjoy that food you've really been craving. Watch the portion size and don't go overboard, but it's better to have a small portion of what you *really* want than to fill up on foods that don't satisfy the urge. Remember, the best way to keep yourself healthy is to do everything in moderation.

COMMONLY ASKED QUESTIONS

I seem to crave certain foods right when I get home from work. My cravings are worse when I've had a stressful day. Am I the only one who experiences this?

No, you're not alone. Almost everyone has cravings, and they tend to be worse during stressful times and/or when you're tired. You may be eating in response to stress, fatigue, or even just because you're hungry! Plan to have a small snack, such as a piece of fruit, some whole-grain crackers, or a small container of low-fat yogurt, before you leave work to help prevent cravings.

I never used to eat sweets but now that I have diabetes, that's all I want to eat. Is this normal?

Many people with diabetes experience those sudden cravings for sweets, particularly when they are first diagnosed.

Why this occurs isn't really known. Sometimes cravings for sweets are a sign that your blood glucose levels are either too high or too low, so it's a good idea to check your blood glucose when the cravings hit. However, the best thing to do is to discuss these cravings with a dietitian who can evaluate your eating plan and even help you fit in foods that you thought you couldn't eat (including sweets).

Summary

Food plays a very important role in everyone's lives. We eat for many reasons, some which are simple, such as plain old hunger, and some which are more complex, including emotions and environmental factors. Pay attention to your cravings and learn what causes you to eat. You may be surprised to find that the answer to dealing with cravings or uncontrolled eating is easy. But if you need help, don't hesitate to talk with a therapist or counselor who specializes in the area of eating disorders. He or she can help you change how you think about and react to food and eating. Finally, remember that food and eating are meant to be enjoyed, and you shouldn't feel guilty if you indulge once in a while, even if you do have diabetes. All foods can fit into anyone's eating plan.

Your Turn

Now it's your turn to recall some key points from this chapter. Let's see how you do!

1. Cravings can be triggered by strict dieting. True or false?

2. Only people with diabetes get cravings. True or false?

3. Waiting 20 minutes before "giving in" to your craving can help the craving subside. True or false?

4. List three triggers that set off your cravings.

   _____

   _____

   _____

5. List three things that you can do to help reduce or eliminate these triggers.

   _____

   _____

   _____

6. Make a list of activities you can do the next time a craving strikes. Post it on your refrigerator, bulletin board, or any place that you can easily see when cravings hit.

See APPENDIX A for the answers.

CHAPTER 16

MAKING FAVORITE RECIPES HEALTHIER

MYTH

People with diabetes should only use diabetic cookbooks and recipes.

SUSAN: I was just diagnosed with diabetes three weeks ago, and I'm still not sure what I can eat. Because I like to cook, I went out and bought some diabetic cookbooks, but to tell you the truth, some of these recipes don't look so good. I don't think my family will like them either, and I'm not looking forward to having to cook two meals—one for me and one for my family—every night.

DIETITIAN: There are actually many excellent cookbooks on the market for people with diabetes. However, having diabetes doesn't mean you have to get rid of all your favorite recipes or cookbooks.

SUSAN: But all my regular cookbooks have recipes that contain sugar and what seems like a lot of fat. I thought I was supposed to cut these things out of my diet.

DIETITIAN: You don't have to stop eating sugar and fat; that's not realistic or even possible. But it's true that many cookbooks have recipes that are too high in fat. I can teach you how to modify your favorite recipes to be lower in both fat and sugar without sacrificing the flavor.

SUSAN: That sounds great! You mean I can still make my famous macaroni and cheese recipe for my family and myself?

DIETITIAN: Sure, and you won't even have to cook different meals for you and for your family. Your meals will taste good, and the only difference is that they'll now be healthier for all of you.

THE OLD AND THE NEW

When was the last time you counted all of the cookbooks on your bookshelf? If you're like Susan, you have probably built up quite a collection over the years, ranging from Fannie Farmer to the latest low-fat, low-sodium, low-carbohydrate diabetic cookbook. Today, there are literally thousands of cookbooks to be found in bookstores and cooking stores across the country. Even more, an endless supply of recipes can be found on the Internet with a click of your computer mouse. In fact, there are so many recipes and cookbooks out there that you may find it overwhelming, especially if you have diabetes. Some cookbooks, of course, are more helpful than others. At the end of this chapter, we'll give you some suggestions for recommended cookbooks to help you out. However, the real purpose of this chapter is to teach you how to modify or change your existing recipes to make them a little lower in fat, sodium, and sugar.

Think back to when you found out you had diabetes. You were likely told that you had to learn many different things, such as how to take insulin or diabetes pills, how to monitor your blood glucose, and how you should eat. Maybe you asked your dietitian or doctor for special "diabetic" recipes or cookbooks, thinking that you could no longer whip up your delicious food creations any more. Or, if one of your family members was diagnosed with diabetes, perhaps you felt compelled to stop preparing many of the traditional family favorites and forgo flavor for dishes that didn't taste quite so good, but were at least "diabetic-friendly."

Luckily, all of that has changed today. The nutrition guidelines for diabetes have changed the way people with diabetes can eat, and for the better. For example, sugar is no longer off limits, because we now know that sugar is a carbohydrate, just like starchy foods (see Chapters 2 and 3). Those infamous "diabetic diets" are now obsolete because there is no such thing as a diabetic diet anymore. Instead, you might be given an eating plan, or guide, to help you make better food choices. Although it's probably smart to keep an eye on your fat and sodium intake, you don't always have to eat bland low-fat, low-sodium foods all the time. Remember: everything in moderation! People with diabetes should be eating the same as people without diabetes, incorporating nutrition principles from the 2005 Dietary Guidelines for Americans. In other words, if you or a family member has diabetes, you do not need to eat any differently from the rest of your family, as long as everyone eats healthfully.

HERE ARE THE FACTS

There are plenty of wonderful cookbooks out there intended for people with diabetes. The good ones include healthy, tasty recipes that don't require a lot of special ingredients (including artificial sweeteners) and provide nutritional information, such as carbohydrate and fat grams, for each recipe. Another marker of a good diabetes cookbook is that the recipes should be geared toward *everyone* in the family, not just the person with diabetes. After all, who wants to prepare two different meals every night? Also, just because a cookbook contains healthful recipes doesn't always mean that they will taste good to you. Taste is very important. If you don't like a particular dish, you'll most likely never make it again.

If you happen to have some older diabetes cookbooks, glance through them. You'll notice that most of the emphasis is on cutting back on or even eliminating sugar. Many of the diabetic recipes include artificial sweeteners or fructose as a substitute for sugar or honey. Although you may still prefer to use artificial sweeteners when cooking, remember that you don't have to completely remove sugar from your recipes. In fact, depending on what you are cooking, sugar is sometimes essential. Baked goods, such as quick breads, cookies, and cakes, require some sugar for leavening, texture, and flavor.

Sugar is a carbohydrate, just like starch. Your blood glucose will rise if you eat too much of *any* kind of carbohydrate, even healthful foods such as breads, pasta, and fruit. Therefore, you don't have to avoid cooking or baking with sugar, but you *do* need to be careful of how much you eat of whatever you are cooking. You may decide to reduce the sugar content in recipes anyway, simply because sugar adds empty calories. In fact, the average American consumes close to 160 pounds of sugar every year. Sugar and sugar-sweetened beverages are linked to obesity and other health problems, so cutting back on you and your family's intake of foods high in sugar is a good idea.

Another major culprit in the American diet is fat. The USDA recommends that we get no more than 35% of our total daily calories from fat. Other institutions and health professionals advocate lower amounts of fat, even as low as 20%. Yet, despite all the messages to lower fat intake, Americans consume about 42% of their calories from fat. Too much dietary fat can lead to many health problems (see Chapter 5). By reducing our fat intake and focusing on eating more vegetables, fruits, and whole-grain foods, we can make a difference in our health and hopefully prevent or delay the onset of major health problems. Although the goal is not to eliminate fat, most recipes can be easily adjusted to be lower in fat and therefore fit in with the dietary guidelines.

Sodium may be a concern for you, especially if you have high blood pressure or congestive heart failure (see Chapter 11). Just as with fat, high-sodium ingredients can be modified in any recipe. If you're concerned about flavor, rest assured that using herbs and spices can substitute nicely for salt.

HERE'S WHAT YOU CAN DO

You don't necessarily need special diabetic cookbooks to cook and eat healthfully. Here are some suggestions that will get you started on modifying your favorite recipes and cooking more healthfully.

1. Learn How to Substitute Ingredients

Thanks to the many lower-fat products available to us, such as nonfat or low-fat milk, cheeses, and margarine, it's relatively easy to make substitutions without dramatically affecting the final taste and texture of a recipe. However, some products work better than others. For example, it's not recommended to cook or bake with fat-free margarine because of its high water content. The same holds true for baking or heating fat-free cheese; you'll end up with a curdled lump of something closely resembling plastic. Fat-free margarine, cheeses, and other dairy foods aren't meant for cooking. In addition, some people find that fat-free foods just don't taste good. If you don't like fat-free mayonnaise or fat-free sour cream, chances are that you won't like the dishes in which you use these items.

Remember that not all fat is bad and that fat carries flavor. You can still use fat in a recipe, just use a little less of it. Or you can decide to trim fat from another meal that day to keep your total fat calories down for the day. Take the time to experiment with different ingredients to find what works and tastes best to you and your family. In the meantime, here are two general rules for baking with less fat and sugar.

1. **Fat.** Use no more than two tablespoons of oil for every cup of flour and slightly increase one of the liquid ingredients to provide enough moistness.

2. **Sugar.** Use no more than 1/4 cup of a nutritive sweetener (sugar, honey, molasses, corn syrup) for every one cup of flour. Reduce the amount of sweetener called for in a recipe by up to one-half the amount.

Ten Tips for Cooking with Less Fat

1. Use fat-free or low-fat milk in place of whole milk.

2. Use reduced-fat cheese or a smaller amount of strong-tasting cheese, such as Romano, sharp cheddar, or blue cheese.

3. Use egg whites or egg substitutes in place of whole eggs.

4. Use lean cuts of red meats, such as top round and tenderloin cuts, trimmed of fat.

5. Remove the skin from chicken and turkey after cooking.

6. Substitute ground turkey or chicken breast for some or all of the ground beef in a recipe.

7. Try "meatless" ground beef, usually made from soy, in place of ground beef.

8. Use canned tuna, salmon, and sardines packed in water, not oil.

9. Use low-fat or light mayonnaise, salad dressings, and tub margarine.

10. Marinate with low-fat salad dressings, flavored vinegars, or fruit juice in place of oil.

---

2. Sweeteners

Many recipes in diabetes cookbooks use non-nutritive, or artificial, sweeteners, such as saccharin, in place of some, or all, of the sugar in the regular recipe. The use of non-nutritive sweeteners can help reduce the calorie content of the recipe as well as the carbohydrate content some-what; however, remember that there will still be carbohy-drate in the food item if there is flour, oatmeal, fruit, etc. You still need to account for this carbohydrate in your meal plan.

The use of non-nutritive sweeteners in baking and cooking is often a matter of individual preference. Now that you know that sugar is no longer off-limits and that you can reduce the sugar content in recipes by half, you may decide not to use non-nutritive sweeteners at all. Some people object to using "chemicals," whereas others simply do not like how they taste. Decide what's best for you. If you choose to use a non-nutritive sweetener, do not automatically eliminate the sugar in the recipe. Sugar is not only there to provide sweetness, it also provides volume, moistness, tenderness, and color. Without sugar, cakes, muffins, and quick breads would be flat, dry, and tough. Non-nutritive sweeteners don't have the same properties as sugar. A good rule is to substitute half of the sugar called for with a non-nutritive sweetener.

There are four sweeteners currently on the market for cooking and baking: saccharin, aspartame, acesulfame-K, and sucralose. The most common brand names, respec-tively, include Sweet 'n' Low, Equal, Sweet One, and Splenda, although there are others. All sweeteners list directions on the box for how to substitute for sugar. Remember, too, that sweeteners are very sweet, so you use much less of them than you would sugar. See Chapter 6 for more information. Here's a quick reference to get you started:

For a 1/4 Cup Sugar, Use

- 6 packets or 1/4 cup of aspartame
- 6 packets or 2 tsp of saccharin
- 6 packets of acesulfame-K
- 1/4 cup sucralose

By the way, using one of these sweeteners in place of 1/4 cup of sugar saves about 190 calories and 50 grams of carbohydrate. If you are baking with sweeteners, it might be wise to choose sucralose, saccharin, or acesulfame-K, although there are now many recipes that use aspartame in baked foods (the aspartame is added at the end of the cooking process and does not break down).

What about other sweeteners, such as honey, molasses, fructose, sugar cane juice, or fruit juice? The bottom line is that sugar is sugar, no matter what the form. If you prefer to use these sweeteners because they are less refined, that's fine, but they still contain calories and carbohydrate. In addition, some recipes don't work well if you use, say, honey in place of sugar. If you want to go ahead with a substitution such as this, first read the recipe or cookbook for special instructions. If those aren't available, pretend you're a food scientist and experiment! You'll never know until you try.

One final word about using less sugar in recipes: if you're concerned that your banana bread or pumpkin pie just won't taste the same without as much sugar, try adding flavorful spices such as cinnamon, nutmeg, or ginger. Extracts, too, can bring out the sweetness in a food; try vanilla, almond, or any other flavor extract.

3. Salt and Sodium

Many people need to cut back on their sodium intake, especially if they have high blood pressure or are prone to retaining fluid. Some people choose to cut back simply to stay healthy. Salt, like fat, provides flavor, so you may be somewhat reluctant to eliminate salt or other high-sodium ingredients from your recipes for fear that it will make your food taste bland and boring. The good news is that you probably have a whole array of flavorful herbs and spices in your cupboard or pantry that work just as well as, if not better than, your saltshaker. On p. 229 are some healthful substitutions for some of the higher-sodium ingredients with which you may normally cook.

In Place Of	Substitute
Salt in recipes	Reduce the amount or use herbs and spices
Baking powder	Low-sodium baking powder
Garlic, celery, or onion salt	Garlic, celery, or onion powder
Bouillon cubes	Low-sodium bouillon granules
Chicken or beef broth	Low-sodium chicken or beef broth
Soy sauce	Reduced-sodium soy sauce
Canned vegetables	Fresh or frozen vegetables or no-salt-added canned vegetables
Canned soups	Reduced-sodium canned soups

In addition to these substitutions, consider mixing up your own blend of herbs and spices to have handy whenever you are cooking. Here's one developed by the American Heart Association.

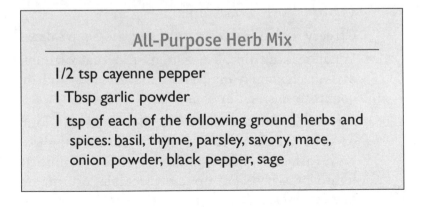

All-Purpose Herb Mix

1/2 tsp cayenne pepper

1 Tbsp garlic powder

1 tsp of each of the following ground herbs and spices: basil, thyme, parsley, savory, mace, onion powder, black pepper, sage

If you don't care for a particular herb, simply substitute it with one you do like. You can even concoct your own herb and spice blends or refer to cookbooks for ideas. To make things easier for you, purchase pre-made herb and seasoning blends, such as Mrs. Dash, right in your grocery store. If you prefer fresh herbs instead of dried ones, the amount you need of a fresh herb will be larger than what you would need if you used the dried version. Use a three-to-one ratio, which means you use one tablespoon of a fresh herb instead of one teaspoon of a dried herb. Once again, adjust the amount to please your taste buds.

4. Lower-Fat Cooking Methods

Okay, you've mastered the substitutions for higher-fat, higher-sodium ingredients. Now you use nonfat milk in recipes, and you've practically eliminated salt from your cupboard. Great! There's still one other topic we need to talk about: ways to cook and prepare foods with less fat without sacrificing flavor. It can be done.

For Salads and Appetizers

- As mentioned previously, use lower-fat salad dressings, make your own with vinegar and less oil, or simply splash on balsamic vinegar, red wine vinegar, or lemon juice for flavor.

- Make your own cream-style dressings with low-fat yogurt or low-fat mayonnaise.

- Go easy with olives, croutons, and cheese in salads.

- When making dips, use nonfat or low-fat versions of sour cream, cream cheese, mayonnaise, and/or yogurt to slash fat and calories.

- Serve dips with homemade tortilla chips (cut flour or corn tortillas into triangles, sprinkle lightly with Parmesan cheese, and broil in the oven until lightly browned); cut-up raw vegetables or fruit; or low-fat crackers.

For Soups

- If you have some time, make your own chicken, beef, or vegetable stock. When making chicken or beef stock, chill or freeze the stock several hours (or even overnight) before you use it. The fat will rise to the top and then you can remove it with a ladle.
- When using canned stocks or broth, whenever possible, buy the lower-fat, lower-sodium versions.
- Cream-style soups don't have to be off-limits. You can find lower-fat versions right on the grocery shelf. A good brand to try is Healthy Choice.
- Use low-sodium bouillon cubes or granules in place of regular bouillon cubes.
- Thicken soups with pureed vegetables, potatoes, or beans. Or make a creamy sauce by mixing a small amount of flour or cornstarch with water or stock, then add to the soup. You can also thicken sauces with this method.

For Main Courses and Vegetables

- Poach fish (and even poultry and red meat) to retain tenderness and moistness.
- Broil or grill meat, poultry, fish, and even vegetables. These methods don't require fat, just flavorful seasonings and careful watching to ensure that your food doesn't burn.
- Bake or roast meat, poultry, or fish in the oven. To prevent sticking, use nonstick roasting pans or lightly spray regular pans with a vegetable oil cooking spray. You can buy pans that allow the grease to drip through a rack and collect in the bottom. Discard the drippings when the food is cooked.
- Try oven-frying your chicken or fish. Dip the food in low-fat batter and bake in the oven at a high temperature. Refer to a heart-healthy cookbook for temperatures and cooking times.

- The next time you make meatballs, consider using ground turkey breast or ask the butcher to grind up the top round cut of beef, which is very lean. Bake your meatballs in the oven instead of frying them. They will brown nicely, and you can pour out the fat before adding them to your sauce.

- Lower-fat stovetop cooking methods include using a nonstick pan, cooking with a vegetable oil cooking spray, and sautéing with water, broth, or wine.

- Stir-frying is another popular cooking method that is fast, easy, and fun. The key is to prepare your ingredients ahead of time, which means chopping the vegetables and meat, poultry, fish, or tofu into small pieces for quick cooking. A wok is ideal for stir-frying, but you can also use a skillet. Use a small amount of vegetable oil, broth, or water for cooking and watch it carefully because foods cook very quickly when stir-frying.

- Invest in a steamer basket to prepare foods without fat and to retain valuable nutrients. You can usually steam any vegetable, as well as fish, in about 10 minutes.

- Don't forget about your microwave. It's not just for popping popcorn or reheating foods. Microwaves are ideal for cooking vegetables and other foods, such as pasta, rice, and even bacon. (Try turkey bacon as a low-fat alternative to regular bacon.)

- If you can't stand the pressure of cooking, get a pressure cooker. Don't worry; they won't blow up in your kitchen. Today's pressure cookers are safe, reliable, and fast. They're great for cooking stews or bean dishes and can cut down on the cooking time by as much as two-thirds. Now that's a time saver!

- It's not just a crock: crock pots (or slow-cookers) are back. Just put in your ingredients for roasted chicken, stews, soups, or sauces; turn it on; and leave it be for 8–10 hours, depending on the dish.

What could be easier? When you get home from work, your meal is good to go.

- Try at least one meatless meal every week, such as vegetarian chili or bean burritos. Don't forget about tofu, either. Tofu works wonderfully in stir-fried dishes. Meatless meals can add variety, cut back on total fat and saturated fat, and lower your grocery bill.

- Consider making a pasta primavera instead of the traditional pasta with heavy meat and cheese sauces. The vegetables in pasta primavera help reduce the caloric content and add important nutrients and fiber. Just be sure not to be too heavy handed with olive oil.

- Try roasting your vegetables instead of just steaming them. Roasting vegetables in the oven retains nutrients and moisture and caramelizes the vegetables' natural sugars, giving them a subtle sweet flavor. To roast, prepare your vegetables and lightly toss with a heart-healthy oil, such as olive or canola oil. Season with herbs or spices, if desired, and then roast at 450 degrees for about 12–20 minutes, depending on the vegetable. The vegetables should be tender and lightly browned.

5. Recommended Cookbooks

There's a vast array of cookbooks on the market, and you've probably got a few on your kitchen bookshelf, too. Many of these cookbooks are excellent. Unfortunately, we don't have room to list them all here. Below is a list of cookbooks that we've chosen to help you in your quest to cook and eat more healthfully. Not all of these are focused toward those with diabetes, either. Hopefully, after reading this chapter, you will feel more confident in making modifications and substitutions on your own. Remember, you don't have to donate your old cookbooks to the library book sale just because you have diabetes—modify those recipes that you like!

The Diabetes and Heart Healthy Cookbook. American Diabetes Association and American Heart Association. Alexandria, Virginia, American Diabetes Association, 2004.

Diabetic Meals in 30 Minutes—Or Less, 2nd Edition. Robyn Webb. Alexandria, Virginia, American Diabetes Association, 2006.

Holly Clegg's Trim & Terrific Diabetic Cooking. Holly Clegg. Alexandria, Virginia, American Diabetes Association, 2007.

Diabetes Fit Food: Over 200 Recipes from the World's Greatest Chefs. Ellen Haas. Alexandria, Virginia, American Diabetes Association, 2007.

The Joslin Diabetes Quick and Easy Cookbook. Frances T. Giedt and Bonnie S. Polin, PhD, with the Nutrition Services Staff at the Joslin Diabetes Center. New York, New York, Fireside/Simon & Schuster, 1998.

Diabetes Cookbook for Dummies. Alan Rubin, Alison Acerra, and Chef Denise Sharf. New Jersey, Wiley Publishing, Inc., 2005.

COMMONLY ASKED QUESTIONS

How can I bake cakes and cookies with less sugar?

Try reducing the sugar content in recipes by one-third or one-half. Slightly increase one of the liquid ingredients in the recipe to give moistness.

I'm tired of baked chicken. How else can I prepare it?

Consider buying a wok and start stir-frying. It's quick, easy, and healthful. Or get a crock pot and make a chicken stew that will simmer all day and be ready in time for dinner. To avoid dryness, marinate chicken breasts in low-fat salad dressing or a small amount of oil and balsamic vinegar, and then broil, grill, or bake.

I like bean dishes, but it takes forever to soak and cook them. Are there any quicker ways to prepare bean dishes?

You can cook dried beans in a pressure cooker. By doing this, you can cut down the cooking time by up to two-thirds. Another option is to buy canned beans, but be sure to drain and rinse them in a colander first so you can get rid of some of the sodium. Some canned beans now come in lower-sodium versions.

I occasionally cook with bacon, but I know that it is very fatty. Are there any good substitutes?

Try turkey bacon. It contains half the fat of regular bacon. Other good choices are Canadian bacon, which is leaner than regular bacon, or vegetarian "bacon," which is usually made from soy beans.

I have a recipe for a decadent, high-fat cheesecake that I love to make for my family, but I know that it is high in fat. Is there any way I can lower the fat content? It contains cream cheese, sour cream, and eggs.

You can certainly make this lower in fat by altering a few ingredients. First, try low-fat cream cheese. Second, use light sour cream. Third, use egg whites or an egg substitute in place of the eggs. There will still be some fat in this cheesecake but a whole lot less!

YOUR TURN

Now it's your turn to recall some key points from this chapter. Let's see how you do!

1. Because you have diabetes, you have to eliminate all of the sugar in your recipes. True or false?
2. Desserts made with non-nutritive sweeteners are free foods. True or false?

3. List three substitutions from the lists on pages 230–233 that you will try when you bake or cook again.

_____

_____

_____

4. Try your hand at modifying the recipe below. Think about how you can reduce both the fat and sodium content of this recipe.

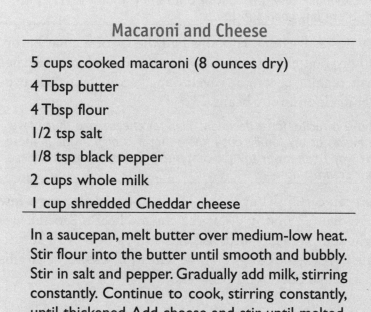

Macaroni and Cheese

5 cups cooked macaroni (8 ounces dry)

4 Tbsp butter

4 Tbsp flour

1/2 tsp salt

1/8 tsp black pepper

2 cups whole milk

1 cup shredded Cheddar cheese

In a saucepan, melt butter over medium-low heat. Stir flour into the butter until smooth and bubbly. Stir in salt and pepper. Gradually add milk, stirring constantly. Continue to cook, stirring constantly, until thickened. Add cheese and stir until melted. In a baking dish, alternate layers of cheese mixture with macaroni. Bake at 350 degrees for 20 minutes until hot and bubbly. Serves 6.

See APPENDIX A for the answers.

"YOUR TURN" ANSWER KEY

CHAPTER 1, PAGE 15

1. medical nutrition therapy
2. true
3.

rice/pasta	1/3 cup cooked
cooked oatmeal	1/2 cup
lentils/beans	1/2 cup
berries	1 cup
milk	8 oz or 1 cup
light margarine/mayo	1 Tbsp
olive oil	1 tsp

4. true

CHAPTER 2, PAGE 28

1. true
2. lactose
3. candy, regular soda, donuts (and others)
4. false

CHAPTER 3, PAGE 41

1. true
2. true
3. soluble
4. fiber

CHAPTER 4, PAGE 57

1. false
2. chicken, fish, eggs (and other meats or dairy products)
3. lentils, tofu, peanut butter (and other beans or soy products)

4. meatless lasagna, beans and rice, soy burgers (and others)

CHAPTER 5, PAGE 71

1. true
2. saturated
3. fat
4. protein
5. protects our major organs
   stores vitamins A, D, E, and K
   prevents dry skin
   intensifies the taste of foods
   maintains our body temperature

CHAPTER 6, PAGE 83

1. false
2. true
3. true
4. aspartame

CHAPTER 7, PAGE 97

1. false
2. 100%, minimal
3. false
4. true

CHAPTER 8, PAGE 115

1. false
2. 130 grams
3. starch or sugar
4. true

CHAPTER 9, PAGE 134

1. true
2. false
3. plate
4. reduce portions, eat less fat, increase physical activity (and others)

5. [answers are based on your own measurements]

Chapter 10, page 150

1. false
2. vitamin C or E, B vitamins
3. true
4. whole-grain breads or cereals, legumes, nuts, bananas, or green leafy vegetables (choose any two)

Chapter 11, page 164

1. 2,300 mg
2. false
3. false
4. don't use the saltshakers, eat fresh or frozen vegetables instead of canned, use fewer high-sodium condiments (and others)

Chapter 12, page 176

1. exercise
2. helps prevent overeating at meals
   continued source of fuel to the body
   helps maintain blood glucose levels when active
3. snacking does not have to cause weight gain
   snacking does not include junk food
   snacking is not being "hungry" between meals
4. true

Chapter 13, page 191

1. better blood glucose control, weight control, lower cholesterol levels (and others)
2. eating a snack before exercising, taking less insulin
3. false
4. start out gradually, exercise with a friend, keep track of my progress (and others)

Chapter 14, page 204

1. plan ahead, take home leftovers, limit alcohol (and others)

2. false
3. grilled
4. true

CHAPTER 15, PAGE 219

1. true
2. false
3. true
4. feeling bored, stress, being told you can't eat a certain food (and others)
5. go for a walk, call a friend, don't keep tempting foods around (and others)
6. [answers will vary]

CHAPTER 16, PAGE 235

1. false
2. false
3. use egg whites instead of whole eggs, use ground turkey breast in place of hamburger, use an herb blend instead of salt (and others)
4. suggestions: use a trans-fat–free tub margarine instead of butter, use half as much salt, use nonfat or low-fat milk, use a reduced-fat cheddar cheese

REGISTERED DIETITIANS AND CERTIFIED DIABETES EDUCATORS

WHAT IS A REGISTERED DIETITIAN?

You may not think there is a difference between a nutritionist and a dietitian, but they are quite different. Here are the facts: any person interested in nutrition can call himself or herself a nutritionist regardless of whether they have had formal training in nutrition. A registered dietitian, however, must have a bachelor's degree from an accredited college or university, complete specific coursework in nutrition and nutrition-related sciences, complete an internship at an accredited institution, and pass a national examination administered by the American Dietetic Association. In addition, every five years, this person must acquire 75 hours of continuing education to remain registered. This ensures that the dietitian has current knowledge of the latest developments and research in nutrition. A registered dietitian will have the credentials "RD" after his or her name, which means that the person has completed academic and experience requirements established by the Commission on Dietetic Registration, an agency of the American Dietetic Association.

What Does a Registered Dietitian Do?

A diabetes educator who is a registered dietitian is uniquely qualified to assess your nutritional needs and establish an eating plan that will meet your individual requirements and goals. Your doctor or health care team may suggest that you meet with this educator for certain conditions or situations, including diabetes and its related health concerns, such as high cholesterol or triglycerides, high blood pressure, overweight or obesity, gastrointestinal disorders, pregnancy, unexplained weight loss, and nutrient deficiency.

Who Should See a Registered Dietitian?

Every person diagnosed with diabetes should receive individualized medical nutrition therapy in order to achieve treatment goals. Although healthy eating is one of the most important tools of diabetes self-management education, studies suggest that many patients with diabetes never receive the recommended instruction but rather get nutrition information from well-intentioned, but misinformed, family and friends. The major share of the responsibility for health maintenance with a chronic disease like diabetes rests with you, but this doesn't mean that you have to go it alone. You and your dietitian need to work together to help you make healthy food choices and change eating behaviors. A dietitian will take into consideration your cultural background, food preferences, and daily schedule to help you form new food behaviors or break unhealthy habits. Registered dietitians are open minded, flexible, and use only realistic approaches to nutrition counseling, which is essential for long-term success.

Where Can I Find a Registered Dietitian?

You can find a registered dietitian in your area by calling your local hospital or by contacting the American Dietetic Association on the Internet (go to www.eatright.org and click on "Find a Nutrition Professional"). In addition, each state has its own dietetic association that can provide you with referrals to dietitians near your home.

What Is a Certified Diabetes Educator?

When you were first diagnosed with diabetes, the person who taught you how to check your blood glucose and how to inject insulin or developed a meal plan for you may have been a Certified Diabetes Educator (CDE). This health professional can also be a nurse, a dietitian, an exercise physiologist, a social worker, a pharmacist, or a doctor. A person who is a CDE specializes in treating and educating people with diabetes. You can find CDEs working in hospitals, outpatient clinics, doctor's offices, pharmacies, and rehab and nursing facilities.

The credentials "CDE" identify a Certified Diabetes Educator. To become a CDE, an eligible health professional must first work in a defined role as a diabetes educator for a specific number of hours for at least two years. After meeting defined eligibility requirements, this person must take and pass a national qualifying examination. The National Certification Board for Diabetes Educators is responsible for the development and administration of this certification program for diabetes educators and is dedicated to promoting excellence in the profession of diabetes education. Every five years, a certified diabetes educator must either take the CDE exam again or renew his or her CDE certification through continuing education.

What Does a Certified Diabetes Educator Do?

CDEs can teach you the skills you need to manage your diabetes. They also have specialized knowledge in diabetes education and a commitment to ensuring that people with diabetes receive the current standards of care. The following types of educators may be part of your diabetes team.

Nurse Educator (RN, CDE)

Nurse educators can teach you diabetes-specific skills, such as how to use and interpret blood glucose meter results and draw up and inject insulin. They can help you understand how your diabetes medication or insulin works and explain how to deal with special situations, such as illness, high and low blood glucose levels, pregnancy, and travel.

Registered Dietitian (RD, CDE)

Dietitian educators have advanced knowledge in meal planning for diabetes. These professionals can give you knowledge of how certain foods or meals may affect blood glucose levels and may teach you how to calculate an insulin dose based on the number of carbohydrate grams you plan to eat. Dietitian educators can help those with special needs—such as children, adolescents, vegetarians. They can also help people who are pregnant, are overweight, are obese, have kidney problems, have high blood pressure, or have high cholesterol levels.

Exercise Physiologist (RCEP, CDE)

Exercise physiologists have specific training to help you learn how to exercise safely. They can teach you how to avoid hyperglycemia and hypoglycemia when you are physically active and can address certain health concerns, such as heart disease, neuropathy, or retinopathy. An exercise physiologist understands these conditions and can prescribe a program that fits your individual needs.

Mental Health Provider

A mental health provider, such as a social worker or a clinical psychologist, can be an indispensable team member who provides support for you and your family. Having diabetes means that you face daily challenges that can often be overwhelming for both you and your loved ones. Meeting with a mental health provider gives you the chance to talk about your concerns and fears about having diabetes, particularly if you are feeling that your diabetes is not well controlled. They can also help you adjust to major lifestyle changes, such as starting a new job, getting married, or dealing with family members without affecting your diabetes self-care.

Where Can I Find a Certified Diabetes Educator?

You can find a CDE in your area by contacting your local hospital or clinic or by contacting the American Association of Diabetes Educators (AADE; a membership organization) on the Internet at www.aadenet.org. You can find an American Diabetes Association Recognized Education Program (a diabetes self-management program that has been recognized by the American Diabetes Association for providing up-to-date standards of care) in your area by contacting 1-800-DIABETES or by visiting them on the Internet at www.diabetes.org.

Index

A

Acceptable Daily Intake (ADI), 76
acesulfame-K, 77, 82
aerobic exercise, 181–183, 215
alcohol, 9, 12, 200–202
American Diabetes Association, 17, 88, 159–160, 190
American Diabetes Association's Medical Nutrition Therapy, 8, 17–20, 61, 74. *See also* medical nutrition therapy
American Dietetic Association, 88
American Heart Association, 8, 159–160
America's Walk for Diabetes, 190
amino acids, 45–46, 49
answer key, 237–240
antioxidant, 139–141, 146, 149
appetite, 212–214
arteries, 67
aspartame, 76–77, 82

B

bacteria, 26
behavior, 131, 215
blood glucose levels, 9, 29–32, 83, 185–188, 200–203
blood pressure, 9, 152–153, 155–159
blood supply, 67
blood vessel disorders, 9
body mass index (BMI), 121–125

C

calcium, 148–149
calories, 23, 25, 67, 101, 105, 126–127
carbohydrate
    complex, 20–21, 32–33, 35
    counting, 31, 86–87, 89–92, 96, 217–218
    definition, 20–23, 106–107
    effects of, 40
    insulin, and, 12–13

carbohydrate (con't)
    Nutrition Facts label, 109–110
    recommendations, 114–115
    serving size, 10–13, 24–27, 175
    simple, 20–21
    sugar substitute, 81–83
    weight loss, 2
cardiometabolic risk, 120
cardiovascular disease, 156
cavities, 26
certified diabetes educator (CDE), 94–96, 184, 243–245.
    See also health care team; registered dietitian
chemicals, 207–208
chloride, 153
cholesterol, 62–66, 106
chromium, 145–146
cinnamon, 146
Consumer Expenditures in 2003, 194
cookbooks, 233–234. *See also* recipes
cortisol, 209
counselor, 219. *See also* health care team; registered dietitian
cravings, 206–219

D
dairy, 11
Davis, Clara, 206
dental caries, 26
diabetes
    education, 14, 211–212
    food recommendations, 88–89
    hyperglycemia, 188
    hypoglycemia, 83, 185–187, 200–203
    treatment, history of, vii–ix. *See also* Old and the New
    type 2, 12–13, 47–48, 119–121
Diabetes Control and Complications Trial (DCCT), 89
Diabetes Prevention Program (DPP), 179
diabetic diet, 5–7
diet
    definition, 1, 211
    diabetic, 5–7
    fad, 53–54, 56
    starvation, 19
Dietary Approaches to Stop Hypertension (DASH), 158
Dietary Guidelines for Americans, 159–160

digestive process, 26
dining out, 162, 195, 197–203
disaccharide, 20–22
disease, heart, 9, 69, 156
disease, kidney, 52–53

E

eating disorders, 214, 219
eating pattern, 167–174. *See also* behavior
education, diabetes, 14, 211–212
education, nutrition
    health care team, 132–133, 150, 214, 219
    registered dietitian, 1–3, 8, 12–14, 27, 94–96
elderly adults, 53, 149
emotions, 213–214
endorphin, 208, 215
entree, 231–233
environment, 214–215
Equal, 76–77, 82
exercise, 2, 131–134, 179–190, 215
    exercise physiologist, 132–133, 184, 187–188, 244. *See also*
    health care team; registered dietitian

F

facts
    cravings, 209–210
    dining out, 194–195
    exercise, 178–179
    food, 2–3, 8–9
    food labels, 103
    meal plan, 89–90
    recipes, 223–225
    snacks, 170–171
    sugar substitute, 75–76
    weight loss, 119
fad diets, 53–54, 56
FAQs (frequently asked questions)
    cravings, 218–219
    eating guidelines, 14–15
    Nutrition Facts label, 114
    recipes, 234–235
    snacks, 174–176
    weight loss, 132–134

fat
    benefits of, 66, 68
    cooking methods, 230–233
    definition, 62, 106
    effects of, 2, 9, 40, 90, 94, 120, 224
    Nutrition Facts label, 109, 112–113
    serving size, 12, 67
    sources, 64–65
    substitutes, 35–36, 226
    weight loss, 128–129, 180
feelings, 213–214
fiber
    benefits of, 35–38, 217
    blood glucose levels, 9, 29–32
    definition, 20–21, 32–35, 40
    glycemic index, 94
    Nutrition Facts label, 109
    recommendations, 38–39
    serving size, 106
    sources, 33–34
    weight loss, 129
food
    exchange, 88, 90–91
    facts, 2–3, 8–9
    glycemic index, 93–94
    guidelines, 9–13, 38–39
    labels, 23–24, 36, 70, 80–83, 101–113, 161
    meal plan, 33–34, 88–90, 130, 187, 196, 216–217
    processed, 153–154
    recommendations, 12–15
    serving size, 11–12
    sugar-free, 82–83
free radicals, 139
fructose, 20–22
fruits, 11, 38, 94

G

galactose, 20–22
galanin, 208
glomeruli, 52
glossary, food label terms, 105–106
glucose, 20–22, 26
glycemic index, 86–87, 89, 92–97
glycogen, 21

grains, 38–39

H

habits, 131, 215
health care team. *See also* nutrition education; registered dietitian
    definition, 241–245
    diabetes education, 14, 211–212
    exercise program, 184, 187–188
health claims, 103
health risks, 15, 48–49, 67, 69, 163, 184–185, 200–201
heart disease, 9, 69, 156
herbs, 229–230
hormones, 208–209
hunger, 212–214
hyperglycemia, 188
hyperlipidemia, 62, 68
hypertension, 156–158
hypoglycemia, 83, 185–187, 200–203

I

identification, 186
ingredients, 103
insoluble fiber, 34–35
insulin, 19, 61, 119–120, 179–180, 186, 202–203
Intersalt Study, 157
isomalt, 82

J

Joslin, Elliot, *Joslin's Diabetic Manual for Doctor and Patient*, 19, 32,
    44–45

K

ketoacidosis, 188
ketone, 188
key, answer, 237–240
kidney disease, 52–53

L

lactose, 20, 22
lipids, 62, 68
lipoproteins, 63–64
liquids, 129, 216

M

magnesium, 144

main course, 231–233

maltodextrin, 36, 82

maltose, 20, 22

meal plan, 33–34, 88–90, 130, 187, 196, 216–217

medical nutrition therapy, 1, 5–8, 17–20, 61, 74, 86–87, 242

medications, 12–14, 163, 187

mental health provider, 244–245. *See also* health care team; registered dietitian

menus, 195, 199

metabolic syndrome, 120

microalbuminuria, 52

minerals, 2, 102, 138–139, 144–150, 153

monosaccharide, 20–22

monounsaturated fats, 64

muscles, 43, 53, 180–181, 183–184

MyPyramid Plan, 127

myths

    diabetic diet, 5–6, 85–86

    dietary supplements, 135–136

    dining out, 193

    exercise, 177–178

    fat, 59–60

    food cravings, 205

    food labels, 99–100

    protein, 43

    recipes, 221–222

    snacks, 165–166

    sodium, 151

    starch, 29–30

    sugar, 17–20

    sugar substitute, 73–74

    weight loss, 117–118

N

National Academy of Sciences Food and Nutrition Board, 97

National Weight Control Registry, 130

neotame, 77

nephropathy, 52–53

neuropeptide Y (NPY), 208

nurse educator, 243–244. *See also* health care team; registered dietitian

NutraSweet, 76–77, 82

nutrients, 101–102, 104–105
nutrition education
    health care team, 132–133, 150, 214, 219
    registered dietitian, 1–3, 8–10, 12–14, 27, 94–96
Nutrition Facts label, 23–24, 80–83, 161
nutrition guidelines, 7
Nutrition Labeling and Education Act of 1990, 101
nutrition recommendations, 1, 5–8, 17–20, 61, 74, 86–87, 242
nutrition science, 1

O

Old and the New
    diabetic diet, 88–89
    dining out, 194
    exercise, 178
    food cravings, 206–207
    food labels, 100–101
    medical nutrition therapy, 7–8
    protein, 44–45
    recipes, 222–223
    snacks, 167–169
    sodium, 152
    starch and fiber, 31–32
    sugar, 18–19
    sugar substitute, 74–75
    vitamins, 136–137
    weight loss, 118
omega polyunsaturated fats, 65

P

physical activity, 2, 131–134, 179–190, 215
Plate Method, 127–128
polydextrose, 36
polysaccharide, 21, 32–33
polyunsaturated fats, 64–65
portion size
    carbohydrate, 24–27, 30, 34, 37
    dining out, 196–198
    fat, 67
    food labels, 101
    foods, common, 10–12
    Nutrition Facts label, 108, 111–113
    protein, 55–56
    restaurants, 202
    weight loss, 127–128, 130

potassium, 163
pregnancy, 149
prehypertension, 156–158
processed food, 153–154
protein
    effects of, 90
    functions, 40, 45
    requirements, 55–57
    serving size, 11–12, 46–49, 175
    sources, 48–51
    weight loss, 2

Q

questions, commonly asked
    cravings, 218–219
    eating guidelines, 14–15
    Nutrition Facts label, 114
    recipes, 234–235
    snacks, 174–176
    weight loss, 132–134
quiz
    answer keys, 237–240
    carbohydrate counting and the glycemic index, 97–98
    cravings, 219–220
    diabetic diet, 15
    dietary supplements, 150
    dining out, 204
    exercise, 191
    fat, 71
    Nutrition Facts label, 115
    protein, 57
    recipes, 235–236
    snacks, 176
    sodium, 164
    starch and fiber, 41
    sugar, 28
    sugar substitute, 83–84
    weight loss, 134

R

recipes, 225–230, 233–234
registered dietitian
    definition, 241–242, 244
    meal plan, 56, 69, 125–126
    nutrition education, 1–3, 8–10, 12–14, 27, 94–96

registered dietitian, conversations with a
    diabetic diet, 5–6, 85–86
    dietary supplements, 135–136
    dining out, 193
    exercise, 177–178
    fat, 59–60
    food cravings, 205
    food labels, 99–100
    protein, 43
    recipes, 221–222
    snacks, 165–166
    sodium, 151–152
    starch and fiber, 29–30
    sugar, 17–18
    sugar substitute, 73–74
    weight loss, 117–118
restaurants, 162, 195, 197–203
Richter, Curt P., 206
roughage. *See* fiber

S

saccharin, 76
SAD (seasonal affective disorder), 207
salt, 9, 106, 153–163, 228–229
"salt sensitivity", 158–159
salt substitutes, 162–163
saturated fats, 65
seasoning, 229–230
serotonin, 207–208
serving size
    carbohydrate, 24–27, 30, 34, 37
    dining out, 196–198
    fat, 67
    foods, common, 10–12
    Nutrition Facts label, 101, 108, 111–113
    protein, 55–56
    restaurants, 202
    weight loss, 127–128, 130
Shaler, Cynthia M., vii–ix
snacks, 2, 171–176, 216–217
sodium, 9, 106, 153–163, 225, 228–229
soluble fiber, 34, 38
soup, 231
Splenda, 77

starch, 20–21, 26, 29–37, 39–40
starvation diet, 19
Step Out to Fight Diabetes, 190
strength training, 183–184
stroke, 156
sucralose, 77
sucrose, 20–23
sugar
    definition, 20–21, 106
    effects of, 9, 224
    myths, 17–20
    Nutrition Facts label, 112–113
    recipes, in, 226
    serving size, 24–27
sugar-free, 106
sugar substitute
    history of, 74–75
    non-nutritive, 76–77
    nutritive, 78–83
    recipes, in, 226–228
    sugar alcohols, 78–83, 107
Sunette, 77, 82
supplements, 2, 102, 137–143, 147–150
support group. *See also* nutrition education; registered
  dietitian
    definition, 241–245
    diabetes education, 14, 211–212
    exercise program, 184, 187–188
Sweet 'n' Low, 76

T

terminology, food label, 105–106
    therapist, 219. *See also* health care team; registered dietitian
tooth decay, 26
trans-fat, 65
treatment, history of diabetes, vii–ix. *See also* Old and the New
Trials of Hypertension Prevention (TOHP II), 157
Trials of Nonpharmacologic Interventions in the Elderly (TONE),
  157–158
triglycerides, 62

U

U.S. Public Health Service, 88
USDA Dietary Guidelines for Americans, 8–9

V

vegetables, 11, 38, 94, 231–233
vitamins, 2, 102, 137–143, 147–150

W

water, 129, 216
weight loss
    blood glucose levels, 2, 7–9
    BMI, 121–125
    calories, 166, 209
    exercise, 180–181
    fad diets, 53–56
    registered dietitian, 14–15
    snacks, 170
Wurtman, Judith, 206–207

The All-Natural Diabetes Cookbook: The Whole Food Approach to Great Taste and Healthy Eating

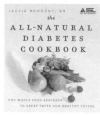

by Jackie Newgent, RD

Instead of relying on artificial sweeteners or not-so-real substitutions to reduce calories, sugar, and fat, *The All-Natural Diabetes Cookbook* takes a different approach, focusing on naturally delicious fresh foods and whole-food ingredients to create fantastic meals that deliver amazing taste and well-rounded nutrition.

Order no. 4663-01; Price $18.95

Diabetes Meal Planning Made Easy, 3rd Edition

by Hope S. Warshaw, MMSc, RD, CDE, BC-ADM

Let expert Hope Warshaw show you how to change unhealthy eating habits while continuing to enjoy the foods you love! This book serves up techniques for changing your eating habits over time so that changes you make are the ones that last for life!

Order no. 4706-03; Price $14.95

The Diabetes Dictionary

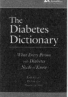

by American Diabetes Association

Diabetes can be a complicated disease; so to stay healthy, you need to understand the constantly growing vocabulary of diabetes research and treatment. *The Diabetes Dictionary* gives you straightforward definitions of diabetes terms and concepts that you need to successfully manage your disease. With more than 500 entries, this pocket-size book is an indispensable resource.

Order no. 5020-01; Price $5.95

Holly Clegg's Trim & Terrific™ Diabetic Cooking

by Holly Clegg

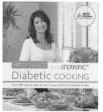

Cookbook author Holly Clegg has teamed up with the American Diabetes Association to create a Trim & Terrific™ cookbook perfect for people with diabetes. With over 250 recipes, this collection is packed with meals that are quick, easy, and delicious. Forget the hassles of meal planning and rediscover the joys of great food!

Order no. 4883-01; Price $18.95

To order these and other great American Diabetes Association titles,
call 1-800-232-6733 or visit http://store.diabetes.org.
American Diabetes Association titles are also available in bookstores nationwide.

The American Diabetes Association is the nation's leading voluntary health organization supporting diabetes research, information, and advocacy. Its mission is to prevent and cure diabetes and to improve the lives of all people affected by diabetes. The American Diabetes Association is the leading publisher of comprehensive diabetes information. Its huge library of practical and authoritative books for people with diabetes covers every aspect of self-care—cooking and nutrition, fitness, weight control, medications, complications, emotional issues, and general self-care.

To order American Diabetes Association books: Call **1-800-232-6733** or log on to **http://store.diabetes.org**

To join the American Diabetes Association: Call **1-800-806-7801** or log on to **www.diabetes.org/membership**

For more information about diabetes or ADA programs and services: Call **1-800-342-2383**. E-mail: **AskADA@diabetes.org** or log on to **www.diabetes.org**.

To locate an ADA/NCQA Recognized Provider of quality diabetes care in your area: **www.ncqa.org/dprp**

To find an ADA Recognized Education Program in your area: Call **1-800-342-2383**. **www.diabetes.org/for-health-professionals-and-scientists/recognition/edrecognition.jsp**

To join the fight to increase funding for diabetes research, end discrimination, and improve insurance coverage: Call **1-800-342-2383**. **www.diabetes.org/advocacy-and-legalresources/advocacy.jsp**

To find out how you can get involved with the programs in your community: Call **1-800-342-2383**. See below for program details.

- American Diabetes Month: educational activities aimed at those diagnosed with diabetes—month of November.
- American Diabetes Alert: annual public awareness campaign to find the undiagnosed—held the fourth Tuesday in March.
- American Diabetes Association Latino Initiative: diabetes awareness program targeted to the Latino community.
- African American Program: diabetes awareness program targeted to the African American community.
- Awakening the Spirit: Pathways to Diabetes Prevention & Control: diabetes awareness program targeted to the Native American community.

To find out about an important research project regarding type 2 diabetes: **www.diabetes.org/diabetes-research/research-home.jsp**

To obtain information on making a planned gift or charitable bequest: Call **1-888-700-7029**. **www.wpg.cc/stl/CDA/homepage/1,1006,509,00.html**

To make a donation or memorial contribution: Call **1-800-342-2383**. **www.diabetes.org/support-the-cause/make-a-donation.jsp**